# THE
# BIG BRAIN
# BOOK

Stephanie Reese, PhD
with Andrew Reese

*We dedicate this book to our patients. We have had the privilege to work with them and to help them change their lives.*

*We also dedicate this book to our children, Christopher, Steven, Elisabeth and Caytlin for whom we started down this path.*

*Finally, we dedicate this book to our grandchildren: Brittney, Makenzie, Tyler, Lexi, Rick, Tyler, Abby, Aiden and Gabriel. If you need us, we're here!*

FOREWORD

INTRODUCTION

# FOREWORD

The brain is the essential generator, source, conduit and projection of everything that we are. It is a complex mini galaxy of neurons and connections that we've only recently been able to explore. Brain imaging has let us learn more about the brain's function in the last twenty years than we did in the previous thousand years. Yet we are just getting started, for the discoveries are accelerating exponentially. There are incredible developments coming, to be sure.

As a neurologist, I have cared for patients with the some of the most debilitating forms of neurological illness. I am excited about the emerging innovations that allow us to salvage damaged nervous systems. And technological advances are allowing us to rescue patients from catastrophic illness with better outcomes than ever before.

But beyond the catastrophic cases I treat every day is a new and exciting frontier, one that this book is all about: neuroplasticity.   Contrary to the old way of thinking, it turns out that the brain can change and reshape itself, provided the user is actively engage in that process.

The long-held belief that the brain was created with a set number of cells that we used (and used up) during our lifetimes has been proven false. We now know that our brains are constantly re-creating themselves. As we learn, new cells and new connections are created. This neuroplasticity, in fact, lets us enhance our brain's performance through our own efforts.

This book should be read by anyone who wants to use their brain better! It is invaluable as a primer for every day brain care. Readers will learn here how to improve their brains' function and thus the quality of their lives. The chapters on nutrition, medication and our environment are particularly valuable, as they present highly relevant material in an easy-to-read presentation.

The Big Brain Book makes the complexity of the human brain understandable and entertaining for those just starting to delve into the world of brain function. The Reeses have brought a large amount of information together in a single volume for a diverse audience, such as thinking professionals, athletes, those with brain-based issues, and for all the rest who just want their brains to function better. And for brain "fans," it provides a glimpse into emerging technologies and exciting new techniques in neurotherapy, all of which will be here before you know it!

Sean C. Orr, M.D.
Neurologist

# INTRODUCTION

The human body is an organic machine composed of a complex network of interconnected systems, each one affecting and being affected by many others. It seems, however, that traditional Western, or allopathic, medicine has forgotten this.

In this post-millennial century, fewer and fewer new medical graduates choose to be general practitioners; the trend is towards specialists with the mindset and training to look only at that part of the body in which they specialize. Today's doctors seem to view the body as a collection of isolated parts that just happen to form a body. Managing such a complex system by fixing an individual component may *sometimes* result in a machine that operates harmoniously. However, the probability is just as great that fixing one part in isolation will interfere with the proper operation of the rest of the body.

Much of allopathic medicine focuses on disease management rather than cure. It frequently uses pharmaceuticals to correct symptoms and address complaints with specific body systems. But when the list of a drug's side effects is longer than the claimed results, something is wrong. The end result is that the root cause of many complaints is never addressed and, as expected, the disease management model does not work to keep anyone in good health.

Now, add in the nutritional deficiencies in the typical American diet and the recent addition of genetically modified foods and you have an American population that is overfed and undernourished. But this has not happened in isolation: we have an industrial society that depends on processing for its profits and treats its waste as a free contribution to nature. Over the past century, we have seen the introduction of a broad range of potent environmental toxins that we only now understand wreaks havoc on our bodies' chemical and electrical systems.

Put it all together—symptom-oriented medical specialization, drug-dominant treatment, rampant dietary deficiencies, pervasive environmental toxins, genetically modified foods—and it's easy to see why we have such trouble staying in good health.

Our health depends on the interrelationships between the nervous, endocrine/hormonal, and immuno systems. These are the control systems that manage the intricate machines that are our bodies. To stay in good health, these systems must work well together and resist the onslaughts from our lifestyles and our environments. In this perfect storm of bodily assaults, brain and body functions fail. With lowered defenses, diseases attack successfully. Even the brain's own processes can go haywire.

Fortunately for us, the human brain has the innate capability to build, patch around, and even heal physical, cognitive, and emotional disturbances. It often needs just a little help to guide it—and the body it controls—back into balance.

The typical allopathic remedy for most brain malfunction has been pharmaceutical chemicals (or if you're *very* unlucky, surgery or electroshock therapy) to treat the symptoms. If a referral is made to another professional, it is often to psychotherapists to examine the social results and potential historical causes of the malfunction. But if the real cause is a brain *functional* issue, it is often ignored. The common answer, then, is to treat the symptom, talk about the problem, but don't consider the true cause.

For issues such as attention deficit disorder (ADHD) and depression, research has shown these pharmaceutical-based interventions are a temporary fix at best. Many times their side effects are far worse than the diseases. By relying upon a pharmaceutical intervention to relieve the symptoms, other significant potential causes are ignored. Allopathic-trained physicians typically ignore poor nutrition, toxic exposures, and the presence of heavy metals in their intake examinations. Vision and auditory processing difficulties are discounted as unrelated. Is it any wonder that the number of people suffering from these neurological disorders keeps increasing?

In the last few years the research community has presented us with an enormous volume of information that has revealed how the brain functions and how it can repair itself. Increasingly powerful imaging systems and brain-affective technology have informed us that the brain is "plastic," i.e., able to change and repair itself *even into old age.*

This revelation that the brain is not a static organ without hope of renewal should be of immense interest to everyone dealing with ADHD, mild cognitive impairment, depression, anxiety, memory loss, traumatic brain injury or even those just wishing to improve brain performance. More than thirty years of research has shown the effectiveness of technology-based neurotherapy. It is non-invasive and virtually free of harmful side effects and enhances brain function while repairing prior damage.

So is there an answer? We think so, but it must begin with knowledge. And that is the intent of this book: to pull together all we have learned about the brain in our decade-plus of research and work with it. You'll find not just the brain and how it works, but also other vital interrelated issues such as nutrition, environmental toxins and medication.

This book is not meant to replace consultation with a medical doctor; it is only intended to be an additional source of information that can help you make intelligent decisions about your body. It is an attempt to provide a glimpse into how the brain and body work together and give you a way to develop a more balanced brain and body through non-invasive means. Hopefully it will illustrate the ways in which we feel that the allopathic mindset is outdated and must be examined by new eyes.

Each of us must recognize the need for safe and effective solutions to brain dysfunction and other diseases—solutions that empower people to be in charge of their inner and outer environments.

# CHAPTER 1
# OUR STORY

Life is learning. Every day you absorb your experiences and the knowledge you gain. Then you file everything away in the recesses of your brain, where it *seems* to disappear completely. At some point later in life, however, you'll be surprised to find it resurface just when you need it—but in a context you never could have contemplated. My life and that of my husband have been shining examples of this.

I worked for 20 years in X-ray and nuclear medicine while my husband was a trial lawyer in northern California. We struggled then with a child with Attention Deficit Disorder, but little was known about it at that time—or even what it was. Most teachers assumed that our son was lazy or that we were inadequate parents. He was referred to a psychiatrist who prescribed drugs without even a follow-up appointment.

We tried him on the drugs and then stopped; he didn't like how he felt when he was taking them, so instead, he learned to cope with his issues.

As our lives evolved, we joined the computer industry in the 1980s and taught art, video production, and 3D modeling and animation in college. We also wrote or edited a number of books on these subjects. I eventually found myself teaching in an elementary classroom while my husband taught a range of disparate subjects in a prep school. What we had learned in our previous work incarnations continued to make appearances in our teaching, either as subject matter or methods.

## FRUSTRATIONS...

My frustrations with teaching in an inner city school finally drove me to start a Ph.D. program in Educational Technology. I thought that with my diverse knowledge and experience, I could create new tools to help children like our son learn more easily. Such schools as the one in which I worked would be ideal to apply these latest advances in educational technology research to better educate young minds.

I hypothesized then that the children in my classes learned differently: they needed extra stimulation to hold their attention. After all, fast-paced video games, *Sesame Street*, and the rapid pace of editing in movies had shaped them to have painfully short attention spans. This appeared to me to require more advanced learning tools than those of our grandparents (or even of our parents or ourselves).

I created new, exciting, visually stimulating activities with a technology base to teach reading to third- through sixth-grade students.

But to my surprise, the children were unable to finish a single task *no matter how exciting the technology*. I struggled with the problem. Why weren't my students able to sustain attention even when the task was fun and exciting?

I began asking questions of my students. All of them qualified for free meals under the National School Lunch Program and 80% spoke Spanish as their primary language. After many discussions, I was amazed to find that *every child in my classroom was taking attention deficit drugs.* They seemed delighted to yell out which medication they were taking. "I'm on Ritalin!" or "I took that, but now I'm on Adderall." It seemed to be a competition to see who was on the "coolest" drug.

There was something drastically wrong with this picture, so I began watching the children more closely. They were 8-to-12 years old and should have been enjoying active lives. I observed their behavior during lunch and at recess.

Their lunches consisted mostly of fat, starch, and sugar. At recess, I noticed that their large motor skills seemed severely underdeveloped. They didn't play as we did as children: no games of tag, four-square, volleyball, tetherball, or football on the field. They stood in groups and talked. Sometimes it seemed that when they did run, they would just run until they came in contact with an immovable object!

I started looking into other aspects of their lives. Nutrition appeared to be an obvious problem. They reported that the only meals they ate were those provided by the school. Many of the parents came to the school for breakfast and lunch as well, as there was not enough food at home for their families.

These meals were very poor nutritionally. A typical breakfast might include a bowl of sugared cereal, a bagel, and a glass of milk. Lunch might include greasy pizza bread and a cookie. The students would bring large bags of Mexican candy to school to keep their hunger in check. If the parents had a few extra dollars, McDonalds® was their restaurant of choice. The school program may have kept these people alive, but did not do them any favors nutritionally.

Many of the children lived in single-parent homes in which the parent worked many hours. For these kids, there were no sports, dance lessons, or other extracurricular activities after school. They spent most of their time watching their siblings while their parents worked. For recreation at home, they occupied their time watching television or playing video games.

Interestingly, although there was little food in the house, these kids seemed to have the best and most up to-date video games and computers: instant gratification provided by the parents to add excitement to their otherwise pretty dismal existences.

To compound the problems suffered by these kids, many of them also lacked a regular sleep schedule. Add sleep deprivation to their already poor nutrition, throw in attention deficit drugs, and many of these students simply fell asleep in class each day.

During this time period, our school received an Intel® Teach to the Future grant. (This program is now a part of their Teach program). I served on the grant committee and acted as liaison to Intel. The grant was a godsend to the school and its students. Intel provided computers and a new lab creating a state-of-the-art teaching tool. The engineers at Intel also acted as "buddies" for the school's latchkey kids. They helped with homework, read stories and even brought Christmas gifts.

Intel also provided instructional materials for after-school courses in science and engineering. Even with all the support from Intel, the school was still labeled a "Needs to Improve" school under the No Child Left Behind Act of 2001 (NCLB).

Our school principal continued to search for some means to help raise the children's scores on the Arizona standardized tests. Higher AIMS (Arizona Instrument for Measuring Standards) scores would satisfy the school improvement program requirements and ensure that NCLB funds would continue to flow.

My principal heard of a new program in a neighboring town and sent me to investigate. What I found was new to me and not precisely within my area of expertise—it definitely wasn't typical Intel-powered hardware.

The system I saw was created by Bridges Learning Systems, Inc. It consisted primarily of a physical gym in which students performed coordinative exercises designed to stimulate their brain functions.

An initial test program in this school divided 100 students into two groups, one as a test group and the other as a control group. Each of the children had been previously tested and determined to be two years behind grade level in reading. One group stayed in their classrooms as controls and the other group went through the physical program for 40 minutes, twice a week during one school year.

At the end of the school year, the 50 students who had remained in their classrooms had progressed a typical nine months in reading. The 50 who had gone through the exercise program had advanced two years!

I was thrilled—just think how this program could help my school's students! I went to Intel and told them about the Bridges Learning program. They were amazed as well, and despite the absence of any Intel technology, they offered to pay for all program costs for my school even without the presence of Intel technology. (Kudos to Intel!) Needless to say, I was elated.

I went to my principal with the wonderful news. To my amazement, the response I received was, "Oh, I don't want that. If we send children through it this year, next year they might go to another school. How is that going to help my test scores today? Go find me a computer program."

I couldn't believe it.

## ...AND TRANSITIONS

I finally realized that part of the educational system, at least, wasn't truly concerned about the individual child, but only about their standardized test scores (and the money that flowed from increasing them). At that moment, I knew that I needed to change the focus of my degree, not to mention that of my life.

One of the members of my Ph.D. committee, Dr. Florence Pittman Matusky, introduced me to a friend of hers, an M.D./ M.D. (H) in Scottsdale, Arizona. This

doctor was doing very exciting work with those with ADHD and Autism Spectrum Disorder using nutrition, acupuncture and brain training.
I explained my experiences to her and what I wanted to accomplish in my Ph.D. program. She enthusiastically agreed to become an adjunct professor and serve on my committee.

As time passed and my program progressed, my husband became involved and together we researched all forms of neurotherapy. In addition to his legal background, he is a computer hardware and software expert. We found that there was a huge and extremely promising area of science being totally ignored by most of the country's population, including its physicians and educators.

During this period, our daughter was in a private high school in the Phoenix, Arizona area. She had a friend I'll call Andi, who was having problems in school. The following is Andi's story. Unfortunately, it is a common theme for too many children in this country.

## ANDI'S STORY

*Andi was diagnosed as having ADHD at the age of six. Her father was a physician and made sure she received all the best that allopathic (standard) medicine had to offer. Over the years she was prescribed all known attention deficit drugs hoping to regulate her symptoms. When she did not take her meds, she would become overly active, loud and boisterous. Her voice would boom louder and louder until medication was forced back upon her.*

*As she grew older, she continued to have trouble coping with the medications and her life. She was a charming girl and very talented in many areas. However, she frequently missed school and it was hard for her to fall asleep at night. Once asleep, she found it difficult to awaken in the mornings.*

*She was constantly depressed. Andi was even placed in medical facilities to "regulate her meds," but by age 15, she was no better. At that point she was re-diagnosed as having a bipolar disorder. She was then placed on anti-psychotic drugs, eventually as many as three at once.*

*When she could no longer sleep at night, Andi was also prescribed sleeping medication. At this point, she became even more depressed and suicidal. She began to hallucinate and cut her skin with razor blades. She was ashamed and riddled with guilt at the hurt she sensed she was causing her parents.*

*Her mother brought her into our office for medical and neurological testing. The first day she was asked, "Do you want to get better?" She responded, "No."*

*We were dumbfounded. How could she say that? Finally she said, "I don't remember a time when I wasn't on drugs. I'm afraid of how it will change me."*

*But she agreed to the therapy. She was assessed with medical, behavioral and neurobiological tests. The results were astounding. She had no symptoms of ADHD or bipolar disorder.*

*However, she also no had sensation in her skin over 80% of her body! This was significant, as her response when asked why she had cut her skin, she said, "Sometimes you just have to feel something."*

*The assessments showed that Andi was hyper-sensitive to sound and light. What sounded to everyone else like tiptoeing sounded like thunder to her. It was impossible for her to ignore any external sounds. Her tendency to become increasingly louder when not taking medication was her defense to drown out the world around her.*

*She was also found to be allergic to a variety of foods and in need of amino acids and nutritional supplements. She was placed on a limited diet and given vitamins and indicated supplements. Twelve weeks of neurotherapy were also prescribed to help her to regulate her auditory and visual processing and to enhance her brain's ability to regulate her symptoms. Early on in her treatment, she noted how quickly her depression had disappeared.*

*At the end of twelve weeks, Andi was off all medications and returned to school. She is now 26 years old, just married and working overseas, doing extremely well. She is much better at coping with her life than she ever was before therapy. She says she has been given a second chance at life and she's going to live it to the fullest.*

# THE BIRTH OF BRAINADVANTAGE

Andi's story was only one of many that convinced me that something had to be done for all the children who were being diagnosed and treated for ADHD. The schools were unable or not willing to take the time to look at each individual child and parents did not know that there was an alternative. The answer had to come from outside the educational system.

I completed my Ph.D. in Cognitive Science and Technologies with a focus in neurobiology and neurophysiology and we formed a company called BrainAdvantage, LLC. My husband contributed his considerable expertise in education and technology and his college friend, Don Barrett, added his entrepreneurial and financial acumen. BrainAdvantage incorporated a new integrated neurotherapeutic approach to multiple brain dysfunctions.

Barrett opened a BrainAdvantage office on Hilton Head Island in South Carolina and we were invited to join a medical group in Scottsdale, Arizona. With a holistic approach to ADHD, post-traumatic stress disorder (PTSD), depression, anxiety and brain injury, Andi's story of recovery and rebirth is not an unusual one for us.

We have seen many people in our practice in similar circumstances. So once again, life has come full circle. We are working to educate the general public as well as skeptical professionals that, yes, these therapies are beneficial to those with brain-based issues like Andi who feel helpless and hopeless. We are doing our part on this quest to make them aware of the alternatives and to give them the opportunity to choose an effective treatment without harm to themselves or the environment.

Ours is truly a sustainable, green, organic and effective medicine. When we look back on the path our lives have taken, we can see a natural progression. There were some leaps along the way, but every day we can see the influence of what we have learned in our daily work. And we continue to learn with each new patient we see.

With the leaps sometimes come surprises. The first surprise was the speed that neurotherapy worked for those with brain-based issues. In one way, this was an expected outcome since we had been doing research on these technologies for several years. On the other hand, we were amazed that our work was effective against so many conditions.

Our clients came with everything from traumatic brain injuries to attention deficit disorder and depression to Parkinson's disease. But very soon something odd started to happen, yet another surprise: our patients were finding that not only did they receive help with their main issues, they were also reporting gains in other areas of their lives that we hadn't anticipated.

Patient after patient reported improvement in sports, business and even musical performance. Athletes reported feeling that events moved more slowly for them, letting them think faster with more accurate responses. Motorcycle riders reported more control on the track, snowboarders had more control of their boards, and divers had better scores; even pianists played with more fluidity.

We knew we needed to look at this a little more closely. We conducted a case study of competition springboard divers. In only a few sessions they all reported improved performance. At 20 sessions, their coach reported their abilities to perform more complex dives with higher quality. Their scores improved across the board. They all had improved their ability to maximize performance.

This book has come from our realization that what we do is not limited only to clinical issues but also has an amazing potential to help "well brains" become even better. It is our attempt to give back some of what we have learned over the long journey to BrainAdvantage. Please use it as it serves your needs.

# CHAPTER 2
# HOW THE
# BRAIN WORKS

*Our right hemisphere is all about this present moment. It's all about "right here, right now." Our right hemisphere thinks in pictures and it learns kinesthetically through the movement of our bodies. Information, in the form of energy, streams in simultaneously through all of our sensory systems and then it explodes into this enormous collage of what this present moment looks like, what this present moment smells like and tastes like, what it feels like and what it sounds like...*

*Our left hemisphere is a very different place. Our left hemisphere thinks linearly and methodically. Our left hemisphere is all about the past and it's all about the future. Our left hemisphere is designed to take that enormous collage of the present moment and start picking out details, details and more details about those details. It then categorizes and organizes all that information, associates it with everything in the past we've ever learned, and projects into the future all of our possibilities.*

*And our left hemisphere thinks in language. It's that ongoing brain chatter that connects me*

*and my internal world to my external world.
It's that little voice that says to me, 'Hey,
remember to pick up bananas on your way
home. I need them in the morning.' It's that
calculating intelligence that reminds me when I
have to do my laundry.*

*But perhaps most important, it's that little
voice that says to me, 'I am. I am.' And as soon
as my left hemisphere says to me 'I am,' I
become separate. I become a single solid
individual, separate from the energy flow
around me and separate from you.*

—*Dr. Jill Bolte Taylor, author of* <u>My Stroke of Insight</u>

The adult human brain is amazing. At right around three pounds, it is estimated to have *100 billion neurons* with *100 trillion connections*. Many of these connections are formed in response to experiences and activities we have every day of our lives. It's hardly surprising, then, that every brain is unique. With its basic genetic blueprint to build from, it is recreated by every day's experiences and this continues throughout our lives. New activities, new thoughts, new experiences prod the creation of new neurons and new neural connections. When we cease an activity, the connections related to it are eventually pruned away.

Although the brain controls everything we sense and do, our understanding of it has accelerated in the last 10 or 15 years. Most importantly, we are now learning how we can guide changes to it.

The flow of information from our senses can be shaped to control the brain's operations and stimulate growth in regions and functions we favor, and discouraged in regions and functions we disfavor. Efficient ways of thinking and acting can be encouraged and inefficient ways can be discouraged. We are also learning the particular locations in the brain that control other areas; this, perhaps, is the most exciting discovery of all.

There are a number of ways to classify and describe the brain. We can look at it:

- **Anatomically**, i.e., where structures are physically located,
- **Functionally**, i.e., where specific functions are carried out in the brain, or
- **Evolutionarily**, that is, how the brain has evolved over time.

We'll start with the last, because it is the most enlightening in understanding what differentiates humans from other species.

# BRAIN STRUCTURE— THE TRIUNE BRAIN CONCEPT

Neurologist Paul MacLean first posited the concept of the "triune brain" in the 1960s. According to this theory, our brain has three distinct structures, representing three human evolutionary periods. Each of these brain structures act like "...three interconnected biological computers, [each] with its own special intelligence, its own subjectivity, its own sense of time and space and its own memory."[1] These three areas are described as follows:

- REPTILIAN BRAIN—the reptilian brain is the oldest, deepest, and smallest area of the brain. It includes the brain stem and cerebellum and is similar to the brains of present-day reptiles which are dominated by these regions. For this reason, it is often called the "reptilian brain." It controls the autonomic functions, such as breathing and blood flow, directs balance and muscle activity and is deeply involved in human survival responses. For example, the "fight or flight" response originates in this part of the brain. We depend upon the reptilian brain to keep us alive in stressful circumstances—and at the base of things, just to keep us breathing!

- LIMBIC SYSTEM—The limbic system is the next evolutionary layer of our brains, occupying intermediate locations between the earlier reptilian brain and the newer cerebral cortex; this facilitates interconnections between thinking processes and survival instincts. The limbic system is generally thought to include the *amygdala*, the *hippocampus*, *parahippocampal gyrus*, *cingulate gyrus*, *fornix*, *hypothalamus*, and *thalamus*. Depending upon the context and the author making the analysis, the limbic system may also be said to include the *mammillary body*, *pituitary gland*, *dentate gyrus*, *entorhinal cortex*, *piriform cortex*,

---

[1] Ashbrook, J.B, (1992) *Brain, Culture, and the Human Spirit*. Lanham. MD : University Press of America.

*olfactory bulb, nucleus accumbens,* and the *orbitofrontal cortex.*

The limbic system connects to the endocrinal system, the autonomic nervous system and the prefrontal cortex, and "engineers" the responses we identify as emotions. Emotions facilitate relationships, typically found in mammals that care for their young, activities and instincts not seen in reptiles that lay eggs and abandon them to natural selection.

- CEREBRAL CORTEX—the cerebral cortex was the last brain layer to form. It comprises the outermost brain layers, where higher functions are maintained. It makes up 85% of the human brain. It's the most highly developed part of the human brain and is responsible for thinking, perceiving, and producing and understanding language.

The triune brain theory works extremely well to help us understand not only how our disparate brain functions are organized, but also how this organization occurred over millennia. Moreover, understanding the triune brain theory helps us to target change in specific parts of the brain. It makes no sense, for example, to attempt emotional change by managing the functions of the brain stem. Emotions tend to "live" in the limbic system and we can make most effective change in emotional disturbances by working on the limbic system—or the control areas that affect it most directly.

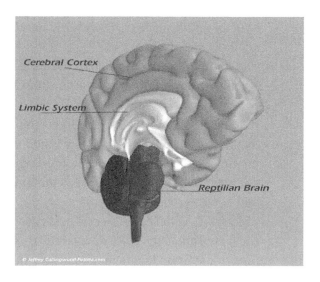

Cerebral Cortex

Limbic System

Reptilian Brain

© Jeffrey Collingwood-Fotolia.com

**Figure 2-1: The Triune Brain**

# Brain Structure— An Anatomical Look

The brain is a collection of structures, all massively interconnected. Three distinct areas can be identified: the forebrain, midbrain and hindbrain.

## Forebrain

The forebrain is the largest portion of the brain. It includes the *cerebrum* (cerebral hemispheres), the limbic system including the thalamus and hypothalamus, and the *corpus callosum* which connects the two hemispheres. Each of the cerebral hemispheres is divided into four lobes: frontal, parietal, occipital and temporal.Frontal Lobe—associated with reasoning, planning, parts of speech, movement, emotions, and problem solving. It includes the prefrontal lobes, involving control of impulses, judgment and decision-making and is the last to mature.

- Parietal Lobe—associated with movement, orientation, recognition, perception of stimuli
- Occipital Lobe—associated with visual processing
- Temporal Lobe—associated with perception and recognition of auditory stimuli, memory, and speech

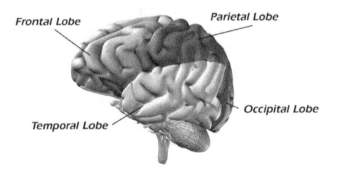

©Andreas Meyer · Fotolia.com

**Figure 2-2: The Forebrain**

Collectively, the forebrain provides cognitive, sensory and motor functions and regulates temperature, reproductive functions, eating, sleeping and the display of emotions.

The largest portion of the brain, the cerebrum, is divided down the middle into completely separate left and right hemispheres, which are inter-connected by a thick band of nerve fibers called the corpus callosum. In general, the left half of the brain controls the right side of the body, and *vice versa*.

In rodents and other small mammals the cerebral cortex is smooth, but in larger primates and humans it has deep grooves (*sulci*) and wrinkles (*gyri*) to increase the surface area of the cerebral cortex considerably without taking up more overall volume. This has allowed humans to evolve new functional areas for enhanced cognitive skills such as working memory, speech, and language.

Motor areas of the cerebrum control muscle movements. Impulses from other brain areas direct such activities as moving the hand muscles for typing or writing and the eye muscles for the physical movement necessary for reading.

Sensory impulses are interpreted in several areas of the cerebrum. In the 1860s and 70s, neurologists Paul Broca and Karl Wernicke observed that when damaged, two specific areas in the left hemisphere resulted in speech and language problems. They noticed that this did not occur with similar damage to the right hemisphere.

These areas of the left hemisphere are now called *Broca's area* and *Wernicke's area*. Wernicke's area translates spoken and written language while Broca's area translates thoughts into speech and coordinates the muscles needed for speaking.

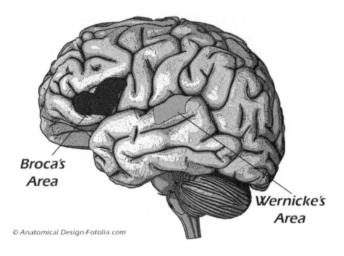

Broca's
Area

Wernicke's
Area

© Anatomical Design-Fotolia.com

**Figure 2-3: Broca's and Wernicke's Areas**

*FUNCTIONS OF THE CEREBRUM*

- Motor movement
- Communication skills,
- Memory
- Ability to learn

*POTENTIAL PROBLEMS WITH THE CEREBRUM*

- Problems with vision and hearing
- Cerebral palsy
- Communication problems
- Seizures

## THE LIMBIC SYSTEM

The limbic system is often referred to as the "emotional brain." It is responsible for both the expression and regulation of emotion. When the deep limbic system is less active, a positive, hopeful state of mind and a neutral or positive interpretation of events are more likely to occur. When it becomes overactive, negativity can increase and dominate.

Using the visual diagnostic technique known as SPECT (Single Photon Emission Computed Tomography), an overactive limbic system can be easily identified as a cause of depression and negativity.

The limbic system and the temporal lobes of the cerebrum have also been reported to store emotional memories, both positive and negative.

If you have been traumatized by a dramatic event, such as being in a car accident or watching your house burn down, the emotional component of the memory is stored in the deep limbic system of the brain. If you have won the lottery, those emotional memories are stored here as well.[2]

The sleep and appetite cycles of the body are also regulated by the limbic system. Healthy sleep and appetite is essential to maintaining a proper internal balance. Limbic abnormalities often cause problems in these areas.

## FUNCTIONS OF THE LIMBIC SYSTEM

- Sets the emotional tone of the mind
- Filters external events through internal states (emotional coloring)
- Tags events as internally important
- Stores highly charged emotional memories
- Modulates motivation

---

[2] Fisher, R. S., Leigh, J. R. & Risinger, M. (2002) Stanford Neurology *Core Clerkship*. CA:Stanford University.

- Controls appetite and sleep cycles
- Promotes bonding
- Directly processes the sense of smell
- Modulates libido

## POTENTIAL PROBLEMS WITH THE LIMBIC SYSTEM

- Moodiness, irritability, clinical depression
- Increased negative thinking
- Negative perception of events
- Decreased motivation
- Flood of negative emotions
- Appetite and sleep problems
- Decreased or increased sexual responsiveness
- Social isolation

## MIDBRAIN

The midbrain is the smallest region of the brain. It provides important connectivity to the auditory, visual and motor systems, as well as producing dopamine, an important neurotransmitter. The degeneration of neurons in the midbrain is often associated with Parkinson's disease.

## FUNCTIONS OF THE MIDBRAIN

- Connectivity for motor functions
- Vision
- Audition (hearing)

## POTENTIAL PROBLEMS WITH THE MIDBRAIN

- Loss of consciousness or coma
- Loss of hearing

- Loss of vision
- Issues with voluntary motor functions

## HINDBRAIN

The hindbrain consists of the *cerebellum*, *pons* and *medulla oblongata*. The pons and medulla are referred to together as the *brainstem* with the medulla immediately connected to the spinal cord and the pons above it connecting to the cerebellum. The medulla can be thought of as a "junction box" between the brain and the spinal cord.

This is the part of the "reptilian brain" that controls the autonomic functions such as breathing, blood circulation, and swallowing. The pons receives and processes visual information, relaying to the cerebellum to maintain body balance and coordination. It also plays a function in sleep regulation.

### FUNCTIONS OF THE HINDBRAIN

- Autonomic processes, such as blood flow, breathing, and swallowing
- Visual processing
- Balance and motor coordination

### POTENTIAL PROBLEMS IN HINDBRAIN

- Stroke
- Sleep disorders
- Balance and coordination difficulties

# Brain Structure— A Functional View

The brain has evolved over time to assign specific functions to specific areas of the brain. These have been researched and verified over generations and if there are no abnormalities, we can be rather certain that a given part of the brain performs a specific function. In some cases, however, this can be changed.

Until William James first proposed the concept of *neuroplasticity* in 1890, the prevailing belief was that you were born with a complement of brain cells, each dedicated to its specific function and unchanging in that function until death. Simply stated, neuroplasticity (or brain plasticity) posits that if a brain injury damages a specific functional area, another area may take over the function. The idea languished from James's initial theory until substantial work was done in the 1960s.

However, it was the basis for a startling revolution in brain science. Scientists now understand that the number of brain cells at any one time is *not* constantly declining but can, in fact, be increased. We have seen remarkable recoveries from brain disabilities through the use of directed brain enhancement.

In the previous evolutionary discussion of brain anatomy, we learned that the deepest parts of the brain are responsible for the least conscious activities. We don't need to think about breathing or keeping our heart pumping or maintaining our balance; all that is handled by the lizard brain (or mid- and hindbrain).

The emotional processing and management of our complex endocrinal system is largely handled by the limbic system with appropriate connections to the cerebrum to associate cognitive activities with emotional content.

In the cerebrum, however, we typically see specific areas perform specific functions. We have seen that Broca's and Wernecke's areas handle specific areas of language processing. Another portion of the cerebrum, the so-called motor strip, directs the actions of our musculature. The occipital lobes process vision signals from the optic nerves. The so-called *executive brain*, across the two frontal lobes behind the forehead, directs many of the other areas of the brain, acting as a decision-maker. In short, each function is handled by a specific area of the brain. See Figure 2-4, below.

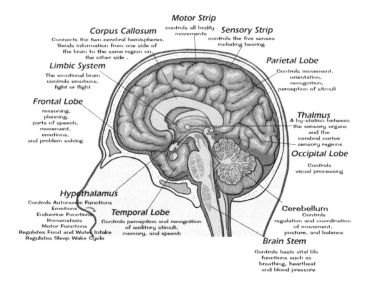

**Figure 2-4: The brain by function**

## NEUROTRANSMITTERS

Each brain cell, or neuron, consists of a cell body with its axon and numerous branching dendrites. Axons typically transmit messages to other brain cells and dendrites receive them. The vehicles for transmitting these messages between cells are a group of chemicals called neurotransmitters. The electrical signal representing a message within a neuron stimulates the production of a neurotransmitter at the axon.

The neurotransmitter passes across the gap (called the synapse) to the target dendrite of a neighboring neuron and is then changed back into an electrical impulse. Then the process begins again. Whenever we act, react, feel emotions, or think, our neurons transmit messages as neurotransmitters, then electrical impulses, and then perhaps as neurotransmitters again. These neural impulses travel across the neural network at an amazing rate of speed—less than 1/5000 of a second to bridge a single synapse. Because they move so quickly, our brains can react almost instantaneously to stimuli such as pain.

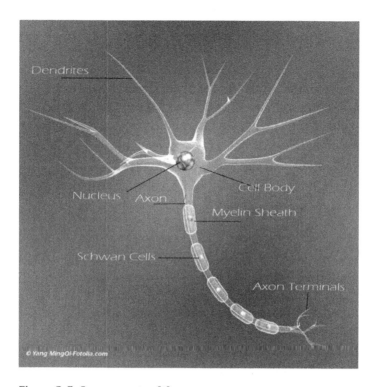

**Figure 2-5: Components of the neuron**

Neurotransmitters travel from neuron to neuron in an orderly fashion creating neuronal pathways. They are specifically shaped so that after they pass from a neuron into the synapse, they can be received by certain sites, called receptors, on the dendrites of a neighboring neuron.

Neurotransmitters can fit a number of different receptors, but receptor sites can only receive specific types of neurotransmitters. Upon landing at the receptor site of a neuron, the chemical message of the neurotransmitter may either be changed into an electrical impulse and continue on its way through the next neuron or it may stop where it is.

These neurotransmitters are also responsible for the regulation of new dendrites to make new connections stimulating plasticity and survival of neurons.

In either case the neurotransmitter released from the receptor site is inactivated in one of two ways. It is either broken down by an enzyme or reabsorbed back into the transmitting neuron that released it. The reabsorption (also known as re-uptake) is accomplished by what are known as *transporter molecules.*

Transporter molecules reside in the cell membranes of the axons that release the neurotransmitters. They pick up specific neurotransmitters from the synapse and carry them back across the cell membrane and into the axon. The reabsorbed neurotransmitters are then available for reuse at a later time.

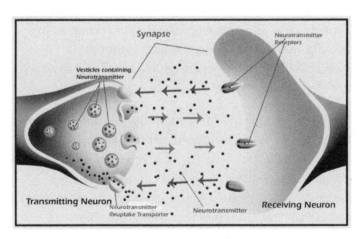

**Figure 2-6: Neurotransmitters transported across a synapse**

# The "Default Brain"

The advent of neuroimaging techniques has allowed us to see brain functions in ways we never have before. PET (Positron Emission Tomography), SPECT and fMRI (Functional Magnetic Resonance Imaging) scanners are all used to image and gauge brain activity.

Think of the brain as a thinking engine that consumes glucose, or blood sugar, as its fuel, and blood oxygen as its oxidizer. At rest, the human brain consumes *20%* of the body's oxygen, even though it is less than *2%* of the body's mass. The glucose and oxygen are made available through the brain's rich network of blood vessels.

In their 2001 paper entitled *Searching for a Baseline: Functional Imaging and the Resting Human Brain,* Debra A. Gusnard and Marcus E. Raichle at Washington University in St. Louis were the first to recognize high activity in the brain even when its owner is daydreaming or wondering *without engaging in any specific mental activity.* [3]

They labeled this the "default mode of brain function." When the person resumed an activity such as memorizing a list of words, a collection of brain regions consistently decreased activity compared to their resting levels. The only time the brain was more active than in the default mode was when recalling autobiographical memories or imagining alternative

[3]Gusnard, D.A.& Raichle, M.E. (2001) Searching for a baseline: functional imaging and the resting human brain. *Nat Rev Neurosci.* 2001 Oct;2(10):685-94.

_Creativity from here?_

situations. Researchers also found even though the brain appeared to be idle, it was using a startling amount of energy.

Raichle hypothesized that the "default brain," has to slow down its activity to allow the brain to focus its energy on a specific task. This phenomenon has been proven through research[4,5,6,7] that suggests that not only is Raichle's hypothesis true, but other more important implications follow.

"It could be running the whole show," said Dr. Ruth Lanius, a neuroscientist at Western University in London, Ont. "It may even be orchestrating all the networks that are active when we engage in cognitive tasks. So this default mode network may serve like a conductor of the whole orchestra that really sets the

---

[4] Fair, D.A., Cohen, A. L., Dosenbach, N. U. F., Church, J., et al. (2008)The maturing architecture of the brain's default network. _Proceedings of the National Academy_ of Sciences 105, 4028-4032. Retrieved from: www.pnas.org/cgi/doi/10.1073/pnas.0800376105

[5] Fair, D.A., Cohen, A. L., Power, J.D., et al. (2009) Functional Brain Networks Develop from a "Local to Distributed" Organization. _PLoS Computational Biology, 5_, e1000381.doi:10.1371/journal.pcbi.1000381

[6] Gao, W., Zhu, H., Giovanello, K.S., Smith, J.K., Shen, D., Gilmore, J.H., & Lin, W. (2009) Emergence of the brain's default network: Evidence from 2-week-old to 2-year-old healthy pediatric subjects. Proceedings of the National Academy of Sciences, 106: 6790-6795 Published online April 7 www.pnas.org/cgi/doi/10.1073/pnas.0811221106

[7] Buckner, R. L., Andrews-Hanna, J. R., & Schacter, D. L. (2008) The Brain's Default Network Anatomy, Function and Relevance to Disease. _Annals of the New York Academy of Sciences, 1124_, 1-38. doi: 10.1196/annals.1440.011

---

brain in what it needs to engage in the future and what it needs to respond to." [8]

The brain's default network may also provide clues to the nature of consciousness. As most neuroscientists acknowledge, our conscious interactions with the world are just a small part of the brain's activity. The brain's default network is always working to interpret information coming into the brain even when we aren't consciously aware. It is critical in providing the context for how we experience our conscious awareness. This network may represent what we experience as our internal monologue and may help generate our sense of self. [9]

The inability to pull one's self out of the default state easily into conscious attention or keep the mind active without slipping back into a default state might also suggest that a malfunctioning default brain might be involved in diseases and disorders such as Alzheimer's disease, attention deficit/hyperactivity disorder, autism, depression and post-traumatic stress disorder.[10]

---

[8] Lanius, R., Bluhm, R., Coupland, N.J., Hegadoren, K.M., Rowe, B., Theberge, J. et al (2010) Default mode network connectivity as a predictor of PTSD symptom severity in acutely traumatized subjects. *Acta Psychiatr Scand* Jan;121(1):33-40.

[9] Fair, D.A., Cohen, A.L., Power, J.D., Dosenbach, N.U. F.,Church, J.A., Miezin, F.M.; Schlaggar, Bradley L.; Petersen, Steven E. (2009). "Functional Brain Networks Develop from a 'Local to Distributed' Organization". In Sporns, Olaf. *PLoS Computational Biology* 5 (5): e1000381. doi:10.1371/journal.pcbi.1000381

[10] Saey, T. H. (2009) Who Are You by Default. *Science News*. Retrieved from: http://www.usnews.com/science/articles/2009/07/08/you-are-who-you-are-by-default

---

Vince Calhoun of the MIND Research Network in Albuquerque and colleagues reported in 2008 in the Proceedings of the National Academy of Sciences that the default system might be faster in people with schizophrenia. [11]

## BRAIN HOMEOSTASIS

Brain Homeostasis is the brain's ability to maintain a stable internal environment. Danger or stress can turn on the fight or flight response, causing a series of stimulating chemicals to be released by the sympathetic nervous system (SNS).

One such chemical is *cortisol*, released by the adrenal glands. Cortisol can be potentially hazardous to the hippocampus, part of the brain's limbic system. Thus, when cortisol is released, the system acts to protect the hippocampus by directing the release of calming hormones which are then rushed to the adrenal glands to suppress the release of cortisol. These hormones allow the cortisol to be flushed through the kidney and bladder.

When the danger has passed and the stress is relieved, the parasympathetic nervous system (PNS) creates a relaxation response and another collection of tranquilizing chemicals are sent from your brain in an attempt to bring you back into balance. This process that brings you back into balance is called *homeostasis*.

---

[11] Swanson, N., Eichele, T., Pearlson, G., Kiehl, K., Yu, Q. & Calhoun, V.D. (2011) Lateral Differences in the Default Mode Network in Healthy Controls and Schizophrenia Patients. Hum Brain Mapp. 2011 Apr;32(4):654-64. doi: 10.1002/hbm.21055.

---

Like a tug-of-war, the SNS and PNS carefully maintain metabolic equilibrium by making adjustments whenever the balance is disturbed. Domination by either the stimulating or tranquilizing chemicals *without relief* produces stress. And this can have serious consequences for your brain.[12]

When stress hormones remain active in the brain for too long, they can injure or even kill cells in the hippocampus, that area of your brain that is intimately involved in memory and learning.

Because of the hierarchical dominance of the SNS over the PNS, it often requires conscious effort to initiate a relaxation response and reestablish metabolic equilibrium.

Bear in mind that an *appropriate* stress response is a healthy and necessary part of life. Stress causes the release of *norepinephrine*, one of the principal excitatory neurotransmitters. Norepinephrine is used to create new memories or improve mood. Problems feel more like challenges, which encourages creative thinking that itself stimulates your brain to grow new connections. [13]Neurotherapy is a tool to create homeostasis in the brain by teaching you how to balance relaxation and stress. Luckily, the brain is able to rebalance itself easily when you know how it's done.

---

[12] Tsigos, C., & Chrousos, G. P. (2002). Hypothalamic -pituitary-adrenal axis, neuroendocrine factors and stress. Journal of psychosomatic research, 53(4), 865–71

[13] Robertson, D. (2004) Primer on the Autonomic Nervous System. (I. Biaggioni & G. Burnstock,Eds.) (second.). San Diego: Elsevier Academic Press.

## A Child's Brain

As a child grows, the brain continues to mature. Several processes occur including *myelination*, an increase in myelin, the insulating covering around the axons. This insulation increases the speed of transmission of nerve impulses within neurons.

Additionally, several important areas of the brain mature, including the corpus callosum which connects the right and left sides of the brain. The prefrontal cortex—that executive brain—increases its authority over other parts of the brain. This improves impulse control and allows children to think before they act as they get older.

As impulsivity decreases and the ability to pay attention increases, children are better able to learn. Young children respond principally through the activity in the limbic system, the amygdala, the hippocampus and the hypothalamus.

- **Amygdala**—develops in early childhood and regulates emotions and fears. Increased activity is one reason for nightmares and night terrors in children. [14]
- **Hippocampus**—lies right next to the amygdala and is the brain's central processor for memory; it responds to anxiety triggered by the amygdala through memories.

---

[14] Berger, M., Gray, J. A. & Roth, B. L. (2009) The expanded biology of serotonin. *Annu. Rev.Med.*, *60*, 355–66. doi:10.1146/annurev.med.60.042307.110802. PMID 19630576

---

- **Hypothalamus**—responds to signals of the amygdala and the hippocampus to produce hormones (including stress hormones) to send to other parts of the brain and body.

All these structures communicate with the prefrontal cortex.

If stress hormones flood the system in infancy and early childhood before the prefrontal cortex has had time to mature, neurons in the hippocampus are destroyed and permanent deficits in learning and memory may occur. [15]

Subjecting children to extreme stress or fear can produce brains that develop abnormally. This can cause a child to be unable to connect emotionally to others, have trouble paying attention, be unable to control impulsivity, and may also demonstrate other emotional issues.

## ARE ATHLETES BETTER AT EVERYTHING?

In March, 2011, The Journal of the American College of Sports Medicine published a study from researchers at the Beckman Institute for Advanced Science and Technology at the University of Illinois at Urbana-Champaign. The study measured whether athletes

---

[15] Fava, G. A., Bernardi , M., Tomba, E. & Rafanelli, C. (2007) Effects of gradual discontinuation of selective serotonin reuptake inhibitors in panic disorder with agoraphobia. *Int. J. Neuropsychopharmacol. 10* (6), 835–8.doi:10.1017/S1461145706007462. PMID 17224089

excel at every task.[16] They recruited 36 male and female students, ages 18 to 22. Half were varsity athletes at the university, a Division I school, and they represented a wide variety of sports, including cross-country running, baseball, swimming, tennis, wrestling, soccer and gymnastics.

Some possessed notable endurance; others, strength and power; and still others, precision and grace. The rest of the volunteers were healthy young collegians but not athletes, from a variety of academic departments.

All used a manual treadmill which was stationed amid three 10-foot-square video screens. One screen stood in front of the treadmill, with the others at either side. Each participant wore goggles that provided an immersive 3D virtual cityscape environment.

When the immersive video began, the students found themselves in an alley between buildings. They were instructed to walk toward a busy street and, once they'd arrived, gauge oncoming traffic. The virtual cars whizzed by in both directions at daunting speeds, a virtual 40 to 55 miles per hour.

When it felt safe, the students were to cross the road. They were told to walk, not run, and had a limit of 30 seconds from the time they left the alley to get to the other side of the road. In some attempts, they had no distractions. In others, they listened to music through

---

[16] Chaddock, L., Neider, M.B., Voss, M.W., Gaspar, J.G. & Kramer, A.F. (2011) Do Athletes Excel at Everyday Tasks? Medicine & Science in Sports & Exercise. doi: 10.1249/MSS.0b013e318218ca74

headphones or chatted on a cell phone with a friend. Each volunteer attempted 96 crossings.

Success varied. The researchers recorded an 85 percent completion rate of participants making it to the other side of the road without incident. The student athletes completed more successful crossings than the non-athletes by a significant margin. This result might be expected considering athletes are typically in peak physical condition.

The interesting fact, however, wasn't that they were quicker than the other participants. They actually didn't walk faster or dive between cars. What they did do, was think faster. They glanced up and down the street more times gathering data and then processed it faster and more accurately than the other participants.

For athletes this seems obvious. In most sports they are required to make split-second decisions. It would then make sense that they would have superior skill sets in processing the fast-paced information to successfully cross the street.

Interestingly, this study was the first to recognize that being adept at sports also allowed success in other area of their lives. Most studies have more narrowly examined parameters and look at whether and why expert athletes are good at athletic activities.

For example, a study published recently by researchers in China found that professional badminton players, when shown video clips of a match, could predict with uncanny accuracy where the shuttlecock would land.[17] Playing elite badminton had made them better able to anticipate what would happen during badminton play.

Would the badminton pros also be capable of navigating crowded city streets better than the amateurs? The new Beckman Institute study would suggest yes. It seems that the constant multitasking and information processing demanded by athletics also increases both the capacity of the athletes' mental information processing systems and their speed.

Although there's always the possibility that these individuals may have been blessed with naturally fine processing abilities and, as a result, became accomplished athletes, the results seem pretty clear that practicing a sport, whether it's running, swimming, tennis or perfecting a back flip, may sharpen your concentration and increase your ability to dodge through a busy intersection without incident.

## MUSCLES AND THE BRAIN

The body contains more than 600 skeletal muscles. Each one consists of thousands of muscle fibers ranging in length from a few millimeters to several centimeters. In order to generate the complex and finely controlled movements that we all take for granted, there has to be a very efficient, fail-safe, and unidirectional transmission between the nerve and muscle fibers that ensures that muscle contractions faithfully follow

---

[17] Jin, H., Xu, G., Zhang, J.X., Gao, H., Ye, Z., Wang, P. et al. (2011) Event-related potential effects of superior action anticipation in professional badminton players. Neurosci Lett. 2011 Apr 4;492(3):139-44. Epub 2011 Feb 12.

commands from the central nervous system.[18] Each muscle fiber is connected to one or more *efferent nerve fibers* (or *motor neurons*) that carry commands from the brain and central nervous system to the muscle, particularly to skeletal muscles. Motor neurons *directly or indirectly control the contraction or relaxation of muscles, which in most cases leads to movement.*

While efferent neurons carry information from the central nervous system to muscles and other systems, *afferent neurons*, or *sensory neurons*, carry information from sensory organs and tissues such as eyes and skin back to the central nervous system.

As we saw earlier in Figure 2-5: Components of the neuron, neurons are composed of three parts: dendrites, cell body and axon. The dendrites branch out from the cell body and receive the electrochemical signals from other parts of the nervous system. The cell body, or soma, contains the necessary cellular components and genetic information needed to keep the cell functional. The axon, or nerve fiber, is considered the most important part of the neuron; the long, thin fiber conducts electrical impulses and sends signals away from the cell to where they are required.

A motor neuron can fall into one of three broad categories.

---

[18] EDWARDS, R. H. T., YOUNG, A., HOSKING, C. P.& JONES, D. A. (1977). Human skeletal muscle function: description of tests and normal values. Clin. Sci. Mol. Med. 52, 283-290.

- Somatic motor neurons are directly involved in the contraction of skeletal muscles and are typically involved in locomotion
- Special visceral motor neurons are involved in the motion of neck and facial muscles
- General visceral motor neurons, sometimes simply called *visceral motoneurons*, are directly involved in the contractions of the heart, the muscles of the arteries, and other viscera (all internal organs in the chest)that are not consciously controlled

Voluntary muscle contraction occurs as a result of conscious effort originating in the brain. The brain sends signals called action potentials through the nervous system to the motor neurons that stimulate the muscle fibers.

In the case of some reflexes, however, the signal to contract can originate in the spinal cord through a communication loop with the grey matter. Involuntary muscles such as the heart or smooth muscles in the gut contract as a result of non-conscious brain activity or stimuli proceeding in the body to the muscle itself.

In humans, motor neurons can only be contracted. In other words, motor neurons cannot directly relax muscles. The relaxation of muscles is caused only by the *inhibition* of motor neurons. [19]

*meditation inhibits motor neurons?*

---

[19] Nikolaidis, M. G.; Kyparos, A.; Spanou, C.; Paschalis, V.; Theodorou, A. A.; Vrabas, I. S. (2012). "Redox biology of exercise: An integrative and comparative consideration of some overlooked issues". *Journal of Experimental Biology* 215 (10): 1615. doi:10.1242/jeb.067470

---

Neuromuscular transmission of these signals depends on the release of the neurotransmitter *acetylcholine*. Acetylcholine is produced by motor neurons and stored in the synaptic vesicles at the terminal end of the axon. When a signal reaches the axon terminal, calcium ions diffuse into the terminal which allows the synaptic vesicles to fuse with the membrane and release acetylcholine. [20]

Acetylcholine is then sent across the neuromuscular junction and is received by the acetylcholine receptors on the muscle fibers cell membrane *sarcolemma*. The sarcolemma is highly folded at the motor end plate to increase the surface area for neurotransmitter reception. This is exactly what is required for voluntary muscles in which a rapid response is required.

The action of acetylcholine is terminated rapidly in about 10 milliseconds. Then an enzyme (*cholinesterase*) breaks the transmitter down into choline and an acetate ion. The choline is then available for re-uptake into the nerve terminal.

---

[20] Faulkner, J. A. (2003). "Terminology for contractions of muscles during shortening, while isometric, and during lengthening". *Journal of applied physiology (Bethesda, Md. : 1985)* **95** (2): 455–459.

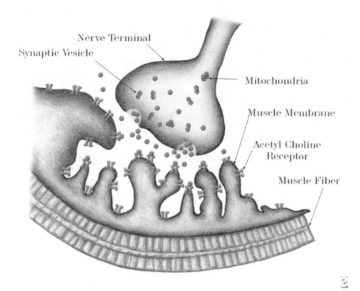

Fig. 2-7

Muscle fibers carry their electrical signals for
contraction on their sarcolemma, the membrane
covering the muscle fiber.[21] Any time that a muscle
fiber has to contract, an electrical signal must run
through its sarcolemma. However, because muscle
fibers have such a large diameter, the electrical signal
is unable to reach the middle of the muscle fiber
quickly.

The sarcolemma is not merely a sleeve over the muscle
fiber. Instead, it tunnels down into the cell, forming
tubes of cell membrane within the muscle fiber. These

[21] Hopkins PM. (2005)Voluntary motor systems—skeletal muscle,
reflexes, and control of movement. In: Hemmings HC & Hopkins PM,
eds. *Foundations of Anesthesia, 2nd edn.* Mosby, London 2005

tubes, called *t-tubules*, are small channels that draw the electrical activity into the depths of the muscle fiber.

Voluntary muscle contraction is controlled by the central nervous system. For the athlete, this means that the brain and nervous system controls the actions of muscles to produce motion. Neurotherapy helps the fluidity of movement and the ability to relax the muscles to enable them to move more efficiently.

# CHAPTER 3
# THYROID AND
# THE BRAIN

*The body's cell membranes are like small batteries, each have measurable voltage. They are made up of opposing phospholipids (fats). Because of their unique properties, this arrangement creates a capacitor, a unit designed to store electrons. Underneath the cell membranes are small power stations called mitochondria. Inside the mitochondria is a rechargeable battery system called ATP/ADP. When the battery is charged, it is called ATP. When it is discharged, it is called ADP. This ATP-ADP cycle controls the storage and use of energy in living things. We have come to understand that chronic disease is accompanied by a loss of voltage at the cellular level.[22]*

Cell mitochondria draw their "fuel" from the *thyroid*, a butterfly-shaped gland in the neck, just above the collarbone. It produces hormones that control how quickly and efficiently cells convert oxygen and nutrients into energy for the cells to use. This chemical activity is known as *metabolism*. Every cell in the body,

---

[22] Tennant, J.L. (2010) *Healing is Voltage: The Handbook*. CreateSpace: Seattle, WA.

including brain cells, depends upon thyroid hormones for regulation of their metabolism.

> *An aside: In lay conversation, the hormones produced by the thyroid gland are often also called "thyroid," as in "Have you taken your thyroid today?" Similarly, a "thyroid test" can be a Thyroid Stimulating Hormone test (or TSH) or it can be a full thyroid panel. The TSH is most often prescribed, but is inherently less accurate; it is used for gross diagnosis only. It should not be relied upon if there is a question about thyroid function. Where the most accurate results are needed, a full thyroid panel should be requested.*

Thyroid hormones are essential for brain development and function throughout life. In adults, thyroid diseases can be the source of many clinical issues.[23]

*Hypothyroidism* (low thyroid hormone level) can cause:

- Lethargy
- Hyporeflexia (low or absent reflexes)
- Poor motor coordination
- Memory impairment
- Bipolar affective disorders
- Depression
- Loss of cognitive functions, especially in the elderly[24]

---

[23] Joffe, R.T. & Sokolov, S.T.H.(1994) Thyroid hormones, the brain, and affective disorders. *Crit. Rev. Neurobiol.* 1994; 8: 45-63.
[24] Ganguli, M., Burmeister, L.A., Seaberg, E.C. et al. (1996) Association between dementia and elevated TSH: a community-based study. Biol. Psychiatr. 1996; 40: 714-725.

*Hyperthyroidism* (high thyroid hormone level) can cause anxiety and irritability. Both conditions, hypothyroidism and hyperthyroidism, can lead to mood disorders such as:

- Dementia
- Confusion
- Personality change

In some patients, hypothyroidism can substantially reduce blood flow and metabolism in parts of the brain. It can also alter the production of brain neurotransmitters whose balance is crucial to normal brain function.

During early brain development, thyroid hormones are required to perform certain actions during specific time frames. Therefore, thyroid hormone deficiencies, even of short duration, may lead to irreversible brain damage, the consequences of which depend on the specific timing of onset and duration of thyroid hormone deficiency.[25]

The longer someone lives with untreated or under-treated hypothyroidism, the more complicated the metabolic abnormalities of body and brain become. As a result of mounting complications, recovering normal body and brain function becomes more difficult. However, full recovery is possible for virtually every patient with diligence. But recovery involves more than merely taking the proper form and dose of thyroid hormone.

---

[25] Bernal J. (2007) Thyroid hormone receptors in brain development and function. *Nat Clin Pract Endocrinol Metab.* 3: 249-259.

# THYROID HORMONES

The thyroid gland converts iodine found in many foods into thyroid hormones. Thyroid cells are the only cells in the body which can absorb iodine. These cells then release the hormones into the bloodstream to be transported throughout the body. Every cell in the body depends upon thyroid hormones for regulation of metabolism.

An underactive thyroid (hypothyroidism) results in reduced cell metabolism of proteins, fats, and carbohydrates. This means not only inefficient transport of nutrients into the cell membrane, but also inefficient transport of wastes out of the cell membrane. Inadequate nourishment and the buildup of toxins (regardless of the cause) in the cells can cause or exacerbate virtually all diseases in the human body. The more the toxins engorge the cells, the more the body becomes susceptible to infections and degenerative conditions.

Interestingly, the mitochondria—the cells' power stations—are intimately affected by thyroid dysfunction.

The hormones secreted by the thyroid include:

- Thyroxine (also known as T4)
- Triiodothyronine (also known as T3)
- T2
- T1

T4 and T3 speed up metabolism and heart rate, thus raising the body's temperature, but T3 is estimated to be anywhere from four to ten times more potent as T4. The normal thyroid gland produces about 80% T4 and about 20% T3, however, T3's metabolic effect is about four times that of T4.

The brain and pituitary gland require freshly converted T3 for their optimal function. It's thought that T4 has little biological activity; its primary role is to serve as source material to be converted into T3 by several target organs, including the brain and liver.

The thyroid also produces *T1* and *T2* hormones. Studies have shown that T2 hormones stimulate metabolism and produce several enzymes needed for proper thyroid gland functioning. At least one study shows that T1 cools the body and slows the heart. Together, all four of these related hormones probably act synergistically in ways that are not yet fully understood.

Thyroid hormones travel through the body linked to protein molecules. T4 and T3 must be first split apart or cleaved from the protein molecules. In its free form, thyroid hormone is known as *free T4* or *FT4* and *free T3* or *FT3*. FT4 and FT3 have biological activity and are able to react with the body's cells.

The typical thyroid hormone level tests prescribed by physicians look at the levels of T4 and T3 hormones. These tests measure the free hormones *together with the protein molecules to which they're linked*. The results may be falsely high or low if the body's stores of binding protein are high or low. Binding protein levels are typically high in pregnancy and in the presence of many medications including estrogens.[26]

# A HYPOTHETICAL PATIENT

Consider a patient whose memory is impaired for several years because she hasn't been treated or she's only been treated with T4. This hormone is most often prescribed by physicians, but is typically less effective than a combination of T3 and T4.

This patient is likely to become frustrated from her struggle to use her hampered short-term memory. Eventually, she may give up trying and find some other way to adapt. She may, for instance, compensate for her poor short-term memory by forming the habit of writing down the most minor things she must attend to—things that most of her life she simply retained in her short-term memory.

After several years of this practice, she'll have become dependent on it. She can recover her capacity for using her short-term memory if she receives proper metabolic and thyroid hormone therapy (often from an alternative doctor), but she may not spontaneously recover the normal use of it. Instead, she may have to retrain herself to use her memory and wean herself from her dependence on note writing.

It is important, then, to consider thyroid function along with other potential causes of low brain function. A

---

[26] Starr, M. (2013) *Hypothroidism, Type 2: The Epidemic.* New Voice Publications: San Diego.

---

complete thyroid panel prescribed by a conscientious physician is the first step toward diagnosing (or eliminating as a cause) thyroid issues. It may also be useful to measure basal body temperature before arising from bed in the morning. This can be an accurate indication of a need for thyroid hormones; discuss this procedure and its indications with your physician.

# Chapter 4
# Oxygen and
# the Brain

Health in the human body depends significantly on how efficiently nutrients can be absorbed and utilized at the cellular level and how efficiently toxins and wastes can be removed from the cells.

Cellular waste can be removed in a variety of ways. Some waste is dissolved in water and transported to the kidneys and liver for filtration and elimination through urine and bowels. Toxins are also excreted from the body through perspiration.

Some of the most toxic poisons, however, can only be neutralized through *oxidation*. Oxidation takes place in the oxygen-rich red blood cells that circulate from the lungs and into the deeper organs and glands of the body. The more oxygen available in the red blood cells and tissues of the body, the better the body will be able to defend itself from toxins and repair damage.[27]

In this chapter we look at some underused and unknown techniques to help improve oxygen in the body and brain.

---

[27] Gesell, Laurie B. (Chair and editor) (2008). *Hyperbaric Oxygen Therapy Indications*. The Hyperbaric Oxygen Therapy Committee Report (12 ed.). Durham, NC: Undersea and Hyperbaric Medical Society.

# OXYGEN BASICS

Oxygen plays a vital role not only in our breathing processes but in every metabolic process in the body. Nutrient compounds inside our cells are oxidized by enzymes and this oxidation process is our main source of energy.

In addition, healthy cells in the body are aerobic, meaning that they require adequate levels of oxygen for cellular respiration and growth. When cells are deprived of oxygen for any reason, decay sets in and cells can mutate or die.[28]

Before it was discovered and isolated, a number of scientists had recognized the existence of a substance with the properties of oxygen. In the early 1500s, Leonardo da Vinci observed that a fraction of air is consumed in respiration and combustion.[29] In 1665 Robert Hooke noted that air contains a substance which is present in potassium nitrate and a larger quantity of an unreactive substance, which we call nitrogen.[21]

By 1668, John Mayow had found that air contained "nitroarial spirit" (the gas oxygen), which is consumed in respiration and burning.[30] Mayow observed that:

- substances do not burn in air from which oxygen is absent

---

[28] Gjedde, A., Poulsen, P. H. & Ostergaard, L. 1999. On the oxygenation of hemoglobin in the human brain. Adv. Exp. Med. Biol. 471:67–81.

[29] Weeks,M.E. (1932) The discovery of the elements. IV. Three important gases. *J. Chem. Educ.* 9 (2), p 215.

[30] Mayow,J. (1674) Tractatus Quinque Medico-Physici, Online Book.

- oxygen is present in the acidic part of potassium nitrate
- animals absorb oxygen into their blood when they breathe
- air breathed out by animals has less oxygen in it than fresh air

Oxygen is utilized by our organs through the simple process of inhaling and exhaling. When we inhale, oxygen we breathe is diffused through membranes in our lungs and into red blood cells. The oxygen-rich blood then circulates throughout the body and finds tissues in need of oxygen.

Enzymes in the body combine with the oxygen molecules and initiate many metabolic processes in the body. One of the waste products is carbon dioxide, which is then released from the cells into the blood when we exhale. It combines with hemoglobin and bicarbonates and is transported back to the lungs— where the process starts again. If your cells need more energy, your breathing rate increases and more oxygen is delivered. If your cells are not receiving enough oxygen, their (and your) energy is decreased.

Oxygen is about 21% of the air we breathe. There is plenty of evidence that our air now contains less oxygen proportionately, especially in densely populated metropolitan areas. Air pollution levels are increasing. Living at higher elevations puts you at an automatic disadvantage—the higher the elevation, the less the oxygen content of the air your breathe.

# OXYGEN AND THE BRAIN

Oxygen is the most vital element to the human body but more important to the brain than to any other organ. While other organs can survive with oxygen deprivation, the brain cannot. Oxygen deprivation in the brain over an extended period can cause coma, seizures, cognitive impairment and even death.[31]

Two pairs of arteries, the internal carotid and vertebral arteries are the main brain blood supply carrying bringing oxygen and glucose to it. The right and left vertebral arteries come together at the base of the brain to form a single basilar artery. The basilar artery joins the blood supply of the internal carotid arteries in a ring at the base of the brain called the *circle of Willis*. It acts as a safety mechanism: if one of the arteries gets blocked, the circle will still provide blood to the brain.[32]

## HYPERBARIC OXYGEN

Hyperbaric Oxygen (HBO) therapy was first documented in 1662, when Henshaw built the first hyperbaric chamber, or "domicilium".[33] By 1877, hyperbaric chambers were used widely for a variety of conditions, although little scientific evidence was available. In 1879, using HBO to prolong safe

---

[31] Sharp, F.R. & Bernaudin, M. (2004) HIF1 and oxygen sensing in the brain. *Nature Reviews Neuroscience* 5, 437-448 (June 2004) | doi:10.1038/nrn1408

[32] Rengachary, S.S. and Ellenbogen, R.G., editors (2005) *Principles of Neurosurgery*, Edinburgh: Elsevier Mosby.

[33] Henshaw N (1664) *Aero-chalinos*. Dublin, Dancer.

anesthesia was found to be effective and was clinically tested. [34]

After WWII, the US military conducted research that showed HBO was effective for such issues as decompression sickness, or "the bends" which occurs if a diver rises to quickly from the depths.[35]

In the 1950s researchers found that an HBO could be used for other clinical issues, but it wasn't until 1962 that the work of Churchill-Davidson and Borema brought HBO treatment into modern medicine.[36]

For the last several years, HBO treatments have been used for a myriad of other issues including wound care[37], traumatic brain injury, and even autism.[38] Today, HBO therapy is being used to help heal and improve symptoms of many conditions, including:

- Non-healing diabetic leg and foot wounds and other selected problem wounds
- Delayed radiation injury to soft tissues (*soft tissue radiation necrosis*)

---

[34] Fontaine, J.A. (1879) Emploi chirurgical de l'air comprime. *Union Med*; 28:445.

[35] Yarbrough, O.D. & Behnke, A.R. (1939) Treatment of compressed air illness utilizing oxygen. *J Indust Hyg Toxicol* 1939; 21:213–18.

[36] Shah, S.A. (2000) Healing with Oxygen: A History of Hyperbaric Medicine. *Pharos Alpha Omega Alpha Honor Med Soc.* 2000 Spring; 63(2):13-9.

[37] Al-Waili, N.S. & Butler, G.J. (2006) Effects of hyperbaric oxygen on inflammatory response to wound and trauma: possible mechanism of action. *Scientific World J* 2006; 6:425-41

[38] Rossignol, D.A. (2010) A Prospective, Randomized, Double-Blind, Controlled Study on the Clinical Effects of Hyperbaric Therapy in Autistic Children, ClinicalTrials.gov Identifier: NCT00335790

- Delayed radiation injury to bone (*Osteoradionecrosis*)
- Compromised skin grafts or flaps
- Carbon monoxide poisoning and smoke inhalation
- Chronic bone infections (*Chronic refractory osteomyelitis*)
- Crush injuries, compartment syndromes, and other acute traumatic injuries
- The "bends" (*Decompression sickness*)
- Necrotizing soft tissue infections
- Gas gangrene (*Clostridial myonecrosis*)
- Serious burn injuries
- Intracranial abscesses
- Air or gas embolisms

The preceding list includes conditions as defined by the Undersea and Hyperbaric Medical Society (UHMS).

## HOW HBO WORKS

Hyperbaric oxygen therapy is a treatment in which a patient intermittently breathes 100% oxygen while the treatment chamber is pressurized to a pressure greater than sea level (1 atmosphere absolute, *ATA*).[39]

The earth's atmosphere normally exerts 14.7 pounds per square inch of pressure at sea level. That is equivalent to one atmosphere absolute (abbreviated as 1 ATA). In this atmosphere, we breathe approximately 20 percent oxygen and 80 percent nitrogen.

---

[39] Hampson, N.B, ed. (1999) Hyperbaric Oxygen Therapy: 1999 Committee report. *Kensington MD, Undersea and Hyperbaric Medical Society*, 1999.

During HBO therapy, the pressure is increased up to twice normal and the patient breathes 100 percent oxygen while the entire body is totally immersed in 100 percent oxygen. Increased pressure combined with the increase in oxygen content dissolves oxygen into the blood and all other body tissues and fluid at up to 20 times the normal concentration.

HBO has complex effects on immunity, oxygen transport and blood flow.[40] The positive therapeutic results include a reduction in hypoxia and edema, enabling normal responses to infection and ischemia.[41]

HBO can also normalize water content in the brain, decrease the severity of brain infarction, and maintain blood–brain barrier integrity. In addition, HBO therapy attenuates motor deficits, and prevents recurrent cerebral circulatory disorders, thereby leading to improved outcomes and survival.

In the treatment of patients with migraine, HBO therapy has been shown to reduce intracranial pressure significantly and abort acute attacks of migraine, reduce migraine headache pain, and prevent cluster headache.[42]

---

[40] Harch, P.G. & Neubauer, R.A. (1999)Hyperbaric oxygen therapy in global cerebral ischemia/anoxia and coma. In: Jain KK ed. Textbook of Hyperbaric Medicine 3d Revised Edition Seattle: *Hogrefe & Huber Publishers;* 1999:319-349.

[41] Knighton DR, Halliday B, Hunt TK. Oxygen as an antibiotic: the effect of inspired oxygen on infection. *Arch Surg* 1984; 119:199–204.

[42] Bennett, M.H., French, C., Schnabel, A., Wasiak, J.& Kranke, P. (2008) Normobaric and hyperbaric oxygen therapy for migraine and cluster headache. *Cochrane Database Syst Rev.* 2008 Jul 16;(3):CD005219

In studies that investigated the effects of HBO therapy on the damaged brain, the treatment was found to inhibit neuronal death, arrest the progression of radiation-induced neurologic necrosis, improve blood flow in regions affected by chronic neurologic disease as well as aerobic metabolism in brain injury, and accelerate the resolution of clinical symptoms.[43]

HBO has also been reported to accelerate neurologic recovery after spinal cord injury by ameliorating mitochondrial dysfunction in the motor cortex and spinal cord, arresting the spread of hemorrhage, reversing hypoxia, and reducing edema. HBO has enhanced wound healing in patients with chronic osteomyelitis.[44,45]

HBO therapy is currently in use for the management of many diseases, and its clinical application is expanding. [46,47] Studies have shown tremendous effects of HBO on nervous system function and disease. The

[43] Rockswold, S.B., Rockswold, G.L. & Defillo A. (2007) Hyperbaric oxygen in traumatic brain injury. *Neurol Res*. 2007 Mar;29(2):162-72.

[44] Asamoto, S., Sugiyama, H., Doi, H., Iida, M.. Naga, O. T., & Matsumoto, K. (2000) Hyperbaric oxygen (HBO) therapy for acute traumatic cervical spinal cord injury. Spinal Cord. 2000 Sep;38(9):538-40.

45 Akin, M.L., Gulluoglu, B.M., Uluutku, H., Erenoglu, C., Elbuken, E., Yildirim, S. et al (2002) Hyperbaric oxygen improves healing in experimental rat colitis. *Undersea Hyperb Med* 2002;29(4):279-85

[46] Shyu WC, Lin SZ, Saeki K, Kubosaki A, Matsumoto Y, Onodera T, Chiang M, et al. (2004) Hyperbaric oxygen enhances the expression of prion protein and heat shock protein 70 in a mouse neuroblastoma cell line. *Cell Mol Neurobiol*. 2004 Apr; 24(2):257-68

[47] Saito, K., Tanaka, Y., Ota, T., Eto, S. & Yamashita, U. (1991) Suppressive effect of hyperbaric oxygenation on immune responses of normal and autoimmune mice. *Clin Exp Immunol* 86(2):322-7

clinical benefits of HBO have been demonstrated in patients with stroke, migraine, headache, elevated intracranial pressure, and brain injury.[48]

It is clear that previous studies have yielded promising results—strong enough to warrant further clinical study of HBO therapy in patients with nervous system disease, particularly stroke, trauma, infection, atherosclerosis, migraine, spinal cord or peripheral nerve injury, and cerebral palsy. [49,50]

## MILD HYPERBARIC OXYGEN

There is a second type of HBO therapy. This is classified as "Mild Hyperbaric Oxygen" (mHBOT). This type of hyperbaric therapy uses an application of pressure less than 1.5 ATA with 100% oxygen. Note that any level of oxygen less than 100% does not constitute hyperbaric oxygen therapy, rather it is identified as *hyperbaric therapy*.

In some case lower pressure is preferable and can be very effective. However, some mHBOT is performed in a lower-cost soft-portable chamber. In our experience, these chambers are inefficient and many times don't deliver the expected results.

---

[48] Veltkamp, R., Siebing, D.A., Heiland, S., Schoenffeldt-Varas, P., et al. (March 2005) Hyperbaric oxygen induces rapid protection against focal cerebral ischemia. *Brain Research* 1037;1-2:134-138 doi:10.1016/j.brainres.2005.01.006

[49] Jain, K.K. (1989) Effect of Hyperbaric Oxygenation on Spasticity in Stroke Patients. *J. Hyperbaric Med* **4** (2): 55–61.

[50] Bouachour G, Cronier P, Gouello JP, Toulemonde JL, Talha A, Alquier P (August 1996). "Hyperbaric oxygen therapy in the management of crush injuries: a randomized double-blind placebo-controlled clinical trial". *J Trauma* **41** (2): 333–9. PMID 8760546

# EXTERNAL COUNTERPULSATION (ECP)

External CounterPulsation (ECP) is a non-invasive therapeutic technique originally designed and used for treatment of angina.[51] ECP is the original acronym, now joined by the acronym EECP® (Enhanced External CounterPulsation) and SECP (Super External CounterPulsation). These are all variants systems that use the same principles. EECP is the registered trademark of Vasomedical, Inc.

ECP is a non-invasive medical system that uses a system of pneumatic cuffs to provide sequential pneumatic compression to the legs and abdomen controlled by a computerized EKG. The compressions are triggered in sequence and inflate and deflate in sync with, but opposite to, the heartbeat.

During the resting phase of the heartbeat, the cuffs inflate beginning the furthest away from the heart and then in sequence toward the heart, pumping oxygen rich blood to the heart and the rest of your body. When your heart beats (pumps), the cuffs rapidly deflate letting the blood vessels expand. The result is that blood gets pumped from the heart with less work for the heart muscle.

ECP works by opening up collateral circulation, "waking up" dormant blood vessels and allowing the

---

[51] Manchanda, A. & Soran, O. (2007) Enhanced external counterpulsation and future directions: step beyond medical management for patients with angina and heart failure. *J. Am. Coll. Cardiol.* 50 (16): 1523–31. doi:10.1016/j.jacc.2007.07.024

blood to bypass or flow around blockages. ECP also creates new blood vessels around the blockages. It does this by releasing VEGF, a growth factor for blood vessels. Amazingly, it also stimulates the bone marrow to produce stem cell endothelial progenitor cells, which create brand new blood vessel cells that line your arteries.

EECP has achieved success rates of 80-90 percent for angina patients providing them relief from chest pain, shortness of breath and fatigue. [52],[53],[54] Increased energy, improved exercise tolerance and less dependency on nitroglycerin were also an added benefit to the treatment. Those doing ECP also had less need for hospitalization, angioplasty, stents and bypass.[55]

So why would we be interested in a heart machine for the brain? The answer lies in understanding that this technique doesn't just affect a simple arterial blockage. It actually is affecting all *60,000 miles* of blood vessels in the body, the entire vascular system from the brain to the toes.

---

[52] Lawson, W.E., Hui, J.C., Soroff, H.S., et al (1992) Efficacy of enhanced external counterpulsation in the treatment of angina pectoris. *Am J Cardiol* 1992; 70: 859-62

[53] Lawson WE, Hui JC, Cohn, PF: Long-term prognosis of patients with angina treated with enhanced external counterpulsation: five-year follow-up study. Clin Cardiol 2000; 23: 254-8

[54] Lawson WE, Hui JC, Oster ZH, et al: Enhanced external counterpulsation as an adjunct to revascularization in unstable angina. Clin Cardiol 1997; 20: 178-80

[55] Arora, R.R., Chou, T.M., Jain, D. et al (2002) Effects of enhanced external counterpulsation on health-related quality of life continue 12 months after treatment: a substudy of the multicenter study of enhanced external counterpulsation. *J Invest Med* 2002; 50: 25-32

ECP not only increases blood flow, but oxygen is increased as it's carried in the red blood cells throughout the body. Increased blood flow and oxygen provides a positive effect in other areas of the body. Peripheral vascular disease, erectile dysfunction, sudden hearing loss and tinnitus, restless leg syndrome, dementia, Alzheimer's disease, Parkinson's disease, stroke, traumatic brain injury, diabetes neuropathy can be improved just to name a few.[56],[57]

[It should be noted that use of ECP for these conditions is "off-label" in that the FDA has only approved it for prescription for these specific conditions: coronary artery disease with angina (chest pain), congestive heart failure, cardiogenic shock, and myocardial infarction. Because the FDA cannot regulate the practice of medicine *per se*, physicians may prescribe ECP for off-label conditions.]

Keep in mind that the flow of blood not only delivers vital substances to the cells, it also "washes out" metabolic debris and environmental toxins. The increased pressure from ECP pumping action drives oxygen and nutrients into cells more effectively. Increased blood flow to kidneys can help flush out toxins and improve function.

The bottom line is that ECP improves blood flow to every organ and cell of the body delivering oxygen and

---

[56] Stys, T., Lawson, W.E., Hui, J.C., Lang, G. et al (2001) Acute hemodynamic effects and angina improvement with enhanced external counterpulsation. *Angiology* 2001; 52: 653-8
[57] Werner,D., Schneider, M., Weise, M., et al (1999) Pneumatic external counterpulsation: A new noninvasive method to improve organ perfusion. The American Journal of Cardiology 1999;84:950-952.

nutrients and removing toxic wastes. It has the potential of preventing vascular diseases and age-related diseases and dementia.

For those suffering from stroke or traumatic brain injury, ECP can improve blood flow to the brain, helping the brain recover more quickly and more completely. It may be the ultimate preventive health maintenance and wellness tool with a profound longevity and anti-aging potential. The treatment is practical, makes sense and can help the body to heal itself. [58]

## WHO SHOULD NOT USE ECP

Although ECP is non-invasive and has been shown to be safe, some people still should not use it. ECP should not be used under the following conditions: pregnancy, severe aortic insufficiency, uncontrolled high blood pressure, abdominal aortic aneurysm, open wounds, deep vein thrombosis (blood clots in legs), hemophilia, high fever.

---

[58] LIN, W., XIONG, L., HAN, J., LEUNG, T.W., SOO, Y.O., CHEN, X., ET AL. (2012) EXTERNAL COUNTERPULSATION AUGMENTS BLOOD PRESSURE AND CEREBRAL FLOW VELOCITIES IN ISCHEMIC STROKE PATIENTS WITH CEREBRAL INTRACRANIAL LARGE ARTERY OCCLUSIVE DISEASE. *STROKE.* 2012 NOV;43(11):3007-11. DOI: 10.1161/STROKEAHA.112.659144. EPUB 2012 SEP 20.

# CHAPTER 5
# THE ENVIRONMENT
# AND THE BRAIN

We have made great technological strides over the last 150 years. Since the Industrial Revolution, we have changed our food, housing, the day-to-day implements we use, the water we drink, our medical practices, even how much we move our bodies.

Beginning with mechanized farming and production, plumbing, electricity, and culminating with today's plastics, computers and engineered foods there have been remarkable achievements. Yet at the same time, it has definitely also been a mixed blessing for our world health. We may live longer than ever before, but we are also learning how our modern lifestyle affects our lives.

The non-biodegradable disposable waste we throw out every day is ending up in our oceans and the toxic remains of our industrialized world are affecting the food we eat, the air we breathe—and our brains.

## ENVIRONMENTAL TOXINS

A huge impact on our life and our environment come from use of chemical cleaning products in our homes. According to the U.S. Environmental Protection Agency (EPA), the average American home generates over 20 pounds of hazardous household waste every year.

Cumulatively, that's *1.6 million tons* or *3.2 billion pounds* of hazardous household waste per year. 176,000 tons alone come from home cleaning products.[59] Yet there is a strange and tragic disconnect between those discarding this waste and the perceived effects on their environments. The Harris Poll found that between January and February 2008, among 1,108 U.S. women over 18 with children under 18 years old still living at home:

- 95% agreed that household cleaning products can be toxic
- 88% agreed that home cleaning products can be harmful to their health and to their families' health
- 61% agreed that the fumes from cleaning products bothered them

Yet 70% of these women thought that home cleaning products were safe to use around their family and only 49% thought that their children may be exposed to household toxins through these chemicals.

And who could blame them? There is little information on the toxicity of 80,000 chemicals registered today with the U.S. EPA.[60],[61] The home cleaning market is

---

[59] EPA (2013) Solid Waste. Retrieved from: http://www2.epa.gov/learn-issues/learn-about-waste.

[60] U.S. Environmental Protection Agency (2009) Statement of Lisa P. Jackson Administrator, U.S. Environmental Protection Agency Legislative Hearing on the Toxic Substances Control Act (TSCA) Senate Committee on Environment and Public Works December 2, 2009 .Retrieved from:
http://yosemite.epa.gov/opa/admpress.nsf/d0cf6618525a9efb852573 59003fb69d/99989761d0557d1d85257680006ff235!OpenDocument

only a small percentage of the chemicals' effects on our environments and our lives.

"Of the 3,000 chemicals produced or imported at over 1 million pounds a year, only 43% have received even minimal toxicological assessment, and a mere 23% have been tested to determine whether they have the potential to cause developmental damage."[62]

According to Dr. Herbert L. Needleman, a University of Pittsburgh pediatrician and who co-authored, *How to Keep Your Child Safe from Lead, Asbestos, Pesticides, and Other Environmental Hazards*, "[w]e are conducting a vast toxicologic experiment in our society, in which our children and our children's children are the experimental subjects." He is right but it's not just one culprit doing damage to our environment and it's not just our environment that's being attacked. It's our bodies and our brains.[63]

## PESTICIDES

Pesticides have been used for centuries to protect crops from insects. In ancient Mesopotamia 4,500 years ago, sulfur dusting was common and by the 15th century, arsenic, mercury and lead were being applied

---

[61] Landrigan, P. J. et al. (2006) U.S. Environmental Protection Agency, New Chemicals Program; The national children's study: a 21-year prospective study of 100,000 American children. Pediatrics, 118(5), 2173-2186.

[62] U.S. Environmental Protection Agency (1998) Chemical Hazard Data Availability Study: What Do We Really Know About the Safety of High Production Volume Chemicals? Washington, DC: U.S. Environmental Protection Agency

[63] Needleman HL, Gatsonis C. 1990. Low level lead exposure and the IQ of children. *J. Am. Med. Assoc.* 263(5):673–78

to crops to kill pests.[64] However in the 1940s, manufacturers began to produce large amounts of synthetic pesticides and their use became widespread.[65],[66]

Pesticide use has increased 50-fold since 1950 and 2.3 million tons of industrial pesticides are now used each year.[67] For nearly three decades DDT, the first synthetic insecticide and an organochlorine, was dominant. It was used to fight malaria, typhus, and the other insect-borne human diseases and for insect control in crop and livestock production, institutions, homes, and gardens. In December of 1972, it was banned in the US when it was found to prevent many fish-eating birds from reproducing.

DDT was replaced in the U.S. by organophosphates and carbamates. It is still used in some countries and, in 2006, the World Health Organization (WHO) gave its approval for indoor use of DDT to fight malaria in countries where the disease remains a major health

---

[64] Miller, G. T. (2002) *Living in the Environment* (12th Ed).. Belmont, CA: Wadsworth/Thomson Learning.
[65] Ritter SR. (2009) Pinpointing Trends In Pesticide Use In 1939. *C&E News*. Retrieved from:
http://pubs.acs.org/cen/coverstory/87/8707cover1a.html
[66] Murphy, G. (2005) Resistance Management — Pesticide Rotation. Ontario Ministry of Agriculture, Food and Rural Affairs. Retrieved from: http://www.omafra.gov.on.ca/english/environment/efp/infosheet_20.htm
[67] Miller G. T . (2004) *Sustaining the Earth*, 6th edition. Pacific Grove, CA: Thompson Learning, Inc.

issue. It was determined by WHO that the disease was worse than the risks of using the insecticide.[68]

Even though the US and many other developed countries banned several pesticides after a 2001 United Nations Convention,[69] other nations aren't required to abide by these domestic bans. [70] Chemicals such as DDT are brought into the US on foreign-grown foods and other produce. Meat, fish and dairy products continue to be the source of most exposure.[71] Over 98% of sprayed insecticides and 95% of herbicides reach a destination other than their target species, including non-target species, air, water and soil.[72]

Originally the majority of pesticides were used primarily in developed countries. More recently, use has increased in developing countries as well.

---

[68] U.S. Environmental Protection Agency (2007) DDT - A Brief History and Status. Retrieved from:
http://www.epa.gov/pesticides/factsheets/chemicals/ddt-brief-history-status.htm

[69] United Nations Environment Programme (2002) Operational Procedures for the Interium Chemical Review Committee Associated with Implementation of the Operational Procedures. *Interium Chemical Review Committee*. Third session, Geneva, 17-21. Feb. 2002, Item 5(b) (v) of the provisional agenda. Retrieved from: *www.pic.int/incs/icrc3/j)/English/ICRC3-9e.pdf*

[70] Fisher, A., Walker, M. & Powell, P. (2006) DDT and DDE: Sources of Exposure and How to Avoid Them. Retrieved from:
http://www.unce.unr.edu/publications/SP03/SP0316.pdf

[71] Center for Disease Control (2009) Prevalence of Autism Spectrum Disorders-Autism and Developmental Disabilities Monitoring Network, United States, 2006. *Morbidity and Mortality Weekly Report, 2009* (58), SS-10.

[72] Miller G. T. (2004) *Sustaining the Earth*, 6th edition. Pacific Grove, CA: Thompson Learning, Inc.

DDT can even be carried on the wind. Over 98% of sprayed insecticides and 95% of herbicides reach a destination other than their target species, including non-target species, air, water and soil.[73] Pesticides are one cause of water pollution, and some pesticides are persistent organic pollutants that contribute to soil contamination.[74]

Behavioral problems and brain damage in young children and fetuses have been linked to many pesticides that are neurotoxins.[75] These pesticides are designed to target the nervous systems of insects.

According to Professor Philippe Grandjean from the Environmental Health Department at Harvard University in Southern Denmark, the human nervous system is similar to that of an insect. Thus, pesticides sprayed to eliminate pests may also harm the human brain.[76]

According to Dr. Patrick Carr and his colleagues at the Energy and Environmental Research Center at the University of North Dakota, there's clear evidence that

---

[73] Miller, G. T. (2002) *Living in the Environment* (12th Ed).. Belmont, CA: Wadsworth/Thomson Learning

[74] Fisher, A., Walker, M. & Powell, P. (2006) DDT and DDE: Sources of Exposure and How to Avoid Them. Retrieved from: http://www.unce.unr.edu/publications/SP03/SP0316.pdf

[75] Landrigan, P. J. et al. (2006) U.S. Environmental Protection Agency, New Chemicals Program; *The national children's study: a 21-year prospective study of 100,000 American children. Pediatrics, 118*(5), 2173-2186.

[76] Grandjean, P. & Perez, M.(2006) *Potentials for exposure to industrial chemicals suspected of causing developmental neurotoxicity.* Boston, MA: Department of Environmental Health, Harvard School of Public Health. Retrieved from: http://www.hsph.harvard.edu/faculty/philippe-grandjean/

pesticide exposure at even relatively low doses can affect human brain cells. When rats are exposed to pesticides Dr. Carr reports, "...some areas of the brain displayed what I would call physical changes—in other words, a loss of neurons in particular regions of the brain. In other regions of the brain you wouldn't notice a change in the number of cells present there, but now the cells that are present there are expressing chemicals in different amounts, compared to normal rats."[77]

In a 2010 study to examine the association between urinary concentrations of dialkyl phosphate metabolites of organophosphates (pesticides) and ADHD in children 8 to 15 years of age, the findings support the hypothesis that organophosphate exposure at levels common among US children may contribute to the prevalence of ADHD. In other words, children who had higher levels of these chemicals in their bodies were more likely to have ADHD symptoms such as impulsivity and attention problems. The link is not absolutely proven by this study, but the evidence is persuasive.[78]

---

[77] University of North Dakota Energy & Environmental Research Center (EERC) (2006) Study of Critical Potential Public Health Risks Related to Pesticide Exposure. Retrieved from:
http://www.newswise.com/articles/view/522287/United Nations Economic & Social Council (1971) United Nations Conference for the Adoption of a Protocol on Psychotropic Substances. Retrieved from: 08/19/09 from http://www.unodc.org/unodc/en/resolution_1971-05-20_1.html

[78] Bouchard,M.F., Sauvé,S., Barbeau,B., Legrand,M., Brodeur,M.E., Bouffard, T. et al (2010) Intellectual Impairment in School-Age Children Exposed to Manganese from Drinking Water. National Institute of Environmental Health Services. doi:10.1289/ehp.1002321 Retrieved from: http://dx.doi.org/

## HEAVY METALS

Heavy metal exposure is also a significant problem. Lead, mercury, aluminum, styrene, tetrachlorobiphenyl, and dioxins are among the neurotoxins that may be airborne and contaminate the air we breathe as well as the food supply.[79] Even though lead paint in America was banned in the 1970s, old buildings with chipping paint can release lead into the environment. Toys and other products imported from other countries that don't ban lead in their manufacture and paint also make their way into our homes and environment.

In the October 2004, the Center for Disease Control estimated that more than 434,000 children between the ages of 1 and 5 had elevated blood lead levels.[80] Lead is also known to be associated with decreased intellectual capabilities and balance disorders among infants, children and teens.[81]

According to Amit Bhattacharya, Ph.D., a professor of environmental health and study collaborator, "We know that lead exposure can affect motor

---

[79] U.S. Environmental Protection Agency (2003) Draft Final Guidelines for Carcinogen Risk Assessment (External Review Draft, February 2003). U.S. Environmental Protection Agency, Risk Assessment Forum, Washington, DC, 2003.Fair, D.A. Dosenbach, N.U.F., Church, J. et al. (2007). Development of distinct control networks through segregation and integration. *Proceedings of the National Academy of Sciences* 104: 13507-13512 www.pnas.org/cgi/doi/10.1073/pnas.0705843104

[80] Center for Disease Control (2006) Summary Health Statistics for U.S. Children: National Health Interview Survey, 2006. Retrieved from: *www.cdc.gov/nchs/data/series/sr_10/sr10_234.pdf*

[81] American Academy of Pediatrics (1998) Screening for Elevated Blood Lead Levels.*Pediatrics,101* (6) 1072- 1078.

coordination—specifically bilateral body coordination (moving arms and legs together), upper limb speed and dexterity, as well as fine motor coordination. But our research shows that this early-life exposure can cause lasting health effects that impact a person's functional abilities well into adolescence and adulthood." [82]

Other toxic contaminants include:

- **Bisphenol A.** This is used primarily in manufacturing of some plastics including baby bottles, water bottles, sports equipment and even coating the inside of all food and beverages cans. In 2007, 38 experts released a statement on bisphenol A concluding that levels of bisphenol A in people were above those that cause harm to animals in laboratory experiments. [83]

  A panel convened by the U.S. National Institutes of Health determined that there was "some concern" about BPA's effects on fetal and infant brain development and behavior. A 2008 report by the U.S. National Toxicology Program (NTP) later agreed with the panel, expressing "some concern for effects on the brain, behavior, and

---

[82] Bhattacharya, A., Shukla, R., Dietrich, K. et al. (2006). Effect of early lead exposure on the maturation of children's postural balance: A longitudinal study. *Neurotoxicology and Teratology*, 28, 376-385.
[83] vom Saal ,F.S., Akingbemi , B.T., Belcher, S.M., et al. (2007) Chapel Hill bisphenol A expert panel consensus statement: integration of mechanisms, effects in animals and potential to impact human health at current levels of exposure. *Reprod. Toxicol. 24* (2), 131–8. doi:10.1016/j.reprotox.2007.07.005. PMID 17768031

prostate gland in fetuses, infants, and children "and that it appeared to alter long-term potentiation in the hippocampus and even a trace dose could induce significant effects on memory processes."[84]

- **Aluminum.** This is one of the most common metals in our environment. It's found in many deodorants and antacids. Despite its natural abundance, aluminum has no known function in living cells and higher concentrations in the body can present some toxic effects. Its toxicity can be traced to deposition in bone and the central nervous system, which is particularly increased in patients with reduced renal function. Because aluminum competes with calcium for absorption, increased amounts of dietary aluminum may contribute to reduced skeletal mineralization (*osteopenia*) observed in pre-term infants and infants with growth retardation. In very high doses, aluminum can cause neurotoxicity, and is associated with altered function of the blood-brain barrier.[85]

- **Industrial emissions.** These emissions are not restricted to the site of an industrial

---

[84] Ogiue-Ikeda, M., Tanabe, N., Mukai, H., Hojo, Y., Murakami, G., Tsurugizawa, T. et al. (2008) Rapid modulation of synaptic plasticity by estrogens as well as endocrine disrupters in hippocampal neurons. *Brain research reviews* , *57*(2), 363–375. doi:10.1016/j.brainresrev.2007.06.010. PMID 1782277

[85] Banks, W. A. & Kastin, A. J. (1989) Aluminum-induced neurotoxicity: alterations in membrane function at the blood-brain barrier. *Neurosci Biobehav Rev* , *13*(1), 47–53. doi:10.1016/S0149-7634(89)80051

---

plant. In fact, a study from researchers at the University of California, Santa Cruz (2002) found that industrial emissions from Asia were a major source of mercury in the rainwater along the California coast.

Although the mercury in rainwater is not in itself a health threat, mercury pollution is a significant problem in the San Francisco Bay and other California waters because the toxic element builds up in the food chain.[86]

## MOLDS

Molds comprise a large portion of the entire range of fungi and are found nearly everywhere on Earth. They can produce reproductive spores that can easily become airborne and spread the contamination throughout an environment. Molds and other fungi can survive in a very wide range of conditions. They are hard to kill, especially where they have grown into substrates, such as wallboard, but they need moisture to grow. These mold spores can enter the air from a hidden mold source with the mere vibration of a stereo or the opening of a door.[87] The toxic mold can then disperse all over a school or home. Once they enter

---

[86] Steding, D., Flegal, R. (2002) Mercury in California Rainwater Linked to Industrial Emissions in Asia; *Media Alerts Archive*, December 19, 2002; Mertl, M. (2000) Running on Ritalin. *Psychology Today, 33*, 5-11.
[87] Kilburn, Kaye H. (2009) Neurobehavioral and pulmonary impairment in 105 adults with indoor exposure to molds compared to 100 exposed to chemicals, *Toxic Ind Health Online First, 2009*, 1-12.

lungs or are swallowed in nasal fluids or saliva, they can travel throughout the body.[88]

The *mycotoxins* produced by toxic mold create environmentally toxic air that depletes the neuron's protective sheath of myelin.[89] The nerves fibers are thus exposed without protection and may malfunction. This affects essential components of the body, including the immune system, the nervous system, the respiratory system, the skin, and the gastrointestinal system.[90]

When toxic mold causes neurological problems, it can be devastating to children, since their brains and other organs are not fully developed.[91] Even a modest exposure can have significant effects.[92] Those who are sensitive to mold need to be extra careful, because they can't remove the toxins from their systems as well as those who are not sensitive to them.

---

[88] Umbach, K.W. & Davis, P.J. (2006) Indoor *Mold; A General Guide to Health Effects, Prevention and Remediation*. Sacramento, CA: California Research Bureau.

[89] Baldo , J. V. et al. (2002) Neuropsychologic performance of patients following mold exposure, *Applied Neuropsychol, 9*, 193-202.

[90] Singer, R. (2005) Clinical Evaluation of Suspected Mold Neurotoxicity, in Bioaerosols, Fungi, Bacteria, Mycotoxins & Human Health: *Proc of the Fifth Int'l Bioaerosal Conference.* 78

[91] Gordon, W. A. et al. (2004) Cognitive impairment associated with toxigenic fungal exposure, *Applied Neuropsychol 11*, 65-74.

[92] Singer, R. (2005) Forensic Evaluation of a Mold (Repeated Water Intrusions) Toxicity Case, 20 ARCHIVES *Clinical Neuropsychol.* , 808.

Mold toxins can result in hundreds of body issues. The following list illustrates some key neurological and psychological findings.[93]

| Headaches | Poor memory | Trouble concentrating |
|---|---|---|
| Trouble Learning | Trouble Finding Words | Disorientation |
| Seizures | Trouble Speaking Fast | Trembling |
| Vocal Or Motor Tics | Serotonin Changes | Abnormal Reflexes |
| Strokes | Edema Or Swelling In The Brain | Scarring Of Brain Seen On MRI's |
| Pet And SPECT Scans Show Hypoperfusion (Low Blood Flow) | Brain And Psychiatric Struggles | Mood Swings |
| Mania | Irritability | Impulsivity |
| Increased Risk Taking | Poor Empathy | Poor Boundary Awareness |
| Immaturity | Spacy (Brain Fog) | Poor Insight |
| Poor Insight Into Illness | Decreased Productivity | Unable To Process Trauma Or Interpersonal Pain |
| Forgetfulness | Poorly Organized or Obsessively Organized | Dead Creativity |
| Depression | Anxiety | Panic Attacks |
| Decreased Attention | Eccentric Personality | Learning Delays |
| Increased Alcohol Consumption Or Increased Drug Use | | |

---

[93] Straus, D., et al. (2004) Studies on the role of fungi in sick building syndrome, pages 83- 86;Kilburn, K. H.,ed. *Molds and Mycotoxins*, Washington, DC: Heldref Publications.

Other symptoms of toxic mold include destruction of brain tissue, open skin sores, fungal infections, lung diseases (such as *Aspergilliosis*), and chronic sinus problems. [94],[95]

## DISORDERS LINKED TO EXPOSURE

There is a growing body of research that suggests that toxic exposure to pesticides, herbicides, lead, aluminum and other contaminates may lead to the death of neurons associated with neurodegenerative diseases such as Alzheimer's, Parkinson's disease, multiple sclerosis, and dementia. A diagnosis of Multiple Chemical Sensitivity has become the center of a new health controversy while disease is a rising occurrence in this country.[96] The diseases linked to toxic exposure highlighted below are only a small sample.

## PARKINSON'S DISEASE

Parkinson's disease is a degenerative disease which is attributed to the deterioration of the *substantia nigra*. The brain structure is located in the midbrain and

---

[94] Singer, R. (2005b) Forensic Evaluation of a Mold (Repeated Water Intrusions) Toxicity Case, 20 ARCHIVES *Clinical Neuropsychol.* , 808.

[95] Kilburn, Kaye H. (2009) Neurobehavioral and pulmonary impairment in 105 adults with indoor exposure to molds compared to 100 exposed to chemicals, *Toxic Ind Health Online First, 2009*, 1-12.

[96] Pall, M. (2005) Multiple chemical sensitivity: towards the end of controversy. Townsend Letter for Doctors and Patients. Retrieved from: http://findarticles.com/p/articles/mi_m0ISW/is_265-266/ai_n15688810/

plays an important role in reward, addiction and movement. As the structure deteriorates, it inhibits production of the neurotransmitter dopamine. As a result, the individual who is suffering from Parkinson's disease will develop symptoms such as tremors, rigidity and instability with sitting and walking.[97]

While we know the *substantia nigra* is the center of Parkinson's disease development not much is known about why the *substantia nigra* begins to inhibit dopamine production or begins to deteriorate. There are some healthcare providers who strongly believe the development of Parkinson's disease may be attributed, in part, to the prolonged exposure to heavy metals. In fact, for individuals with more than 20 years of exposure to heavy metals, there does seem to be a correlation between that exposure and the increased incidence of Parkinson's development.[98]

About 50,000 new cases of Parkinson's disease are reported annually in the U.S. and the prevalence of Parkinson's is expected to double by 2030.[99] In recent studies manganese, cadmium, and nitrogen dioxide as well as herbicides such as Agent Orange and Malathion, a popular organophosphate insecticide, were linked to

---

[97] Jankovic, J. (2008) Parkinson's disease: clinical features and diagnosis. *J. Neurol. Neurosurgery. Psychiatry. 79* (4), 368–76. doi:10.1136/jnnp.2007.131045

[98] Powers, K. M., et al. (2003) Parkinson's Disease Risks Associated with Dietary Iron, Manganese, and Other Nutrient Intakes. *Neurology 60*, 1761–66.

[99] National Institute of Neurological Disorders & Stroke. (2002) Traumatic brain injury: hope through research. Bethesda (MD): National Institutes of Health; 2002 Feb. NIH Publication No.: 02–158.

Parkinson's disease.[100] In 2009, the Institute of Medicine 2008 Veterans Agent Orange biennial review reported that exposures to Malathion and Agent Orange used in Vietnam have a positive association with Parkinson's disease in exposed veterans.[101]

Alberto Ascherio and his colleagues at the Harvard School of Public Health looked at data from roughly 143,000 people involved in a cancer and diet study, of which 413 were diagnosed with Parkinson's disease in the 1990s. They found that those who reported exposure to pesticides had a 70% greater risk of developing Parkinson's disease than those who said they had no such exposure. But exposure to other toxic compounds—such as asbestos and formaldehyde—had no effect on their chances of acquiring the illness.[102]

## ALZHEIMER'S DISEASE

Alzheimer's disease is estimated to affect nearly 4.5 million people in the U.S. About 5% of men and women aged 65–74 have Alzheimer's disease, while nearly half of those aged 85 and older may have the disease. By

[100] Aschner, M., Erikson, K. M., Hernández, E. H. & Tjalkens, R. (2009) Manganese and its Role in Parkinson's Disease: From Transport to Neuropathology. *NeuroMolecular Medicine*, 11 (4), 233-324.
[101] U.S. Veterans with Parkinson's disease (2009) Petition for Presumptive Service-Connection for Parkinson's disease due to herbicide exposures. Letter to Secretary of Veterans Affairs U.S. Department of Veterans Affairs
[102] Ascherio, A., Chen, H., Weisskopf, M.G., O'Reilly, E., McCullough, M.L., Calle, E.E. , et al.(2006) Pesticide exposure and risk for Parkinson's disease. *Annals of Neurology*, 60 (2),197-203.

2050, researchers estimate that this number will nearly triple to over 13 million.[103]

Alzheimer's disease is also among the degenerative illnesses that have been identified as being linked to toxic exposure. A recent study showed 21% of more than a thousand patients presenting to a university clinic for cognitive disorders had medical histories that suggested they may have been exposed to chemicals in their workplace or from an environmental source. Clinicians also found that a history of toxic exposure was associated with cognitive decline at significantly younger ages.[104]

Recent evidence also links environmental lead exposure in the community to increased risk of cognitive impairment. For example, a recent study of elderly men found that the highest lead-exposed group had on average an additional 15 years of cognitive aging, compared to the lowest lead-exposure group. Several animal studies suggest that exposure in infancy and childhood may sharply increase the risk of Alzheimer's disease decades later.[105]

---

[103] National Institute of Neurological Disorders & Stroke (NINDS) (2002) Traumatic Brain Injury: Hope through Research. NIH Publication No. 02-2478 . Retrieved from:
http://www.ninds.nih.gov/disorders/tbi/detail_tbi.htm

[104] Schmechel, D. E., Browndyke, J., & Ghi, A. (2006) Strategies for Dissecting Genetic-Environmental Interactions in Neurodegenerative Disorders, *Neurotoxicology*, *27*(5), 637–57.

[105] Stein, J, Schettler, T., Rohrer, B., Valenti, M., & Meyers, N. (ed) (2008) *Environmental Threats to Healthy Aging*. Boston: Greater Boston Physicians for Social Responsibility and the Science and Environmental Health Network.

Additionally, a recent French study found that a history of occupational exposure to pesticides more than doubled the risk of developing Alzheimer's disease. Exposure to some pesticides has also been linked to dramatically increased risks for diabetes, pre-diabetes, and metabolic syndrome.[106]

Toxic molds have been linked to Alzheimer's disease as well. The effects of toxic mold (*Stachybotrys*) can actually mimic Alzheimer's disease with loss of memory and the ability to think logically.[107] In fact, researchers are starting to recommend that if someone is starting to show signs of Alzheimer's disease, the first step would be to thoroughly mold test the person's home and work environment for the presence of *Stachybotrys*.

Because *Stachybotrys* is rarely airborne, a very thorough physical inspection is necessary, including inside HVAC units, walls, ceilings, floors, attics, crawl spaces, and basements in order to locate mold deposits that should be directly sampled for mold analysis.

If a person is experiencing possible health effects from *Stachybotrys* mold, the first step for that person and all other residents is to leave the home or workplace until thorough mold inspection and mold testing has been completed.

---

[106] Alonzo, P.W. (2008) Pesticide Use Increases Chance of Parkinson's in Men. Retrieved from:
http://www.yourlawyer.com/topics/overview/pesticide_parkinsons_di sease
[107] Kilburn, Kaye H. (2009) Neurobehavioral and pulmonary impairment in 105 adults with indoor exposure to molds compared to 100 exposed to chemicals, *Toxic Ind Health Online First*, *2009*, 1-12.

If *Stachybotrys* does cause brain damage, the brain damage is usually permanent and irreparable.[108]

## COGNITIVE IMPAIRMENT

Two National Institute of Environmental Health Science (NIEHS) researchers, Jean Harry and Jau-Shyong Hong, theorize that environmental exposures have a latent effect on the brain, causing noticeable degeneration years after the fact. As an example, after a stroke, the victim's surviving neurons sprout and make new connections, striving to keep the brain in balance.

As the system ages, however, it gradually loses the ability to compensate, and an accelerated aging process may begin. "You may have been exposed to something when you were five years old," Harry says, "Basically, the whole process sort of catches up with you." Hong and his colleagues in the Laboratory of Toxicology at the NIEHS theorize that microglia, the smallest of the brain's glial cells often referred to as "nurse cells" because they protect neurons, somehow become activated by neurotoxins or other injuries and are suddenly transformed from loyal bodyguards into overactive destroyers. They kill the very neurons they were intended to protect.[109]

---

[108] American Environmental Health Foundation (2003) Innovative Aspects and Treatment of Molds, Mycotoxins and Chemical Sensitivity. *21st Annual International Symposium on Man and His Environment in Health and Disease.*

[109] Harry, J., & Hong, J. S. (1996) Environmental Toxins and the Brain. *Environmental Health Perspectives 104, (8),* 22. Retrieved 09/12/09 from http://www.ehponline.org/docs/1996/104-8/niehsnews.html

When the brain is injured—either through adverse environmental exposure, a viral or bacterial infection, trauma, or stroke—these nurse cells launch an out-of-control rampage in the brain. Hong likens the process to misuse or overuse of a beneficial drug. Too much of a good thing, he says, can be very harmful. "When these glial cells work too hard, they not only kill the foreign invader, they also kill the neurons," he explains.[57]

High levels of lead were also associated with cognitive decline. A 2004 study showed the substantial impact lead is having on cognitive aging across the population. Researchers divided a population of elderly men into four groups, based on the amount of lead found in the bones of their kneecaps. They found that each increasing level of bone lead was associated with accelerated cognitive aging; the group with the highest level of exposure had 15 years of additional cognitive aging compared to the group with the lowest level.[110]

Recent animal studies have resurrected the 1960s controversy about the potential role of aluminum in neurodegenerative disease. One small study showed that when rodents were chronically exposed to dietary aluminum (similar to typical human exposure levels), aluminum accumulated in the brain. A larger follow-up study in rats showed that the more aluminum a rat received in its diet, the more memory loss it exhibited.[111],[112]

---

[110] Weisskopf, M.G., et al. (2004) Cumulative Lead Exposure and Prospective Change in Cognition among Elderly Men, *American Journal of Epidemiology, 160*(12), 1184–93.
[111] Walton, J.R. (2007a) A Longitudinal Study of Rats Chronically Exposed to Aluminum at Human Dietary Levels, *Neuroscience Letters, 412*, 29-33

## MULTIPLE SCLEROSIS

Multiple sclerosis (MS) is a debilitating neurological disorder that strikes more than a quarter of a million people in the United States each year.[113] Multiple sclerosis creates numerous lesions, or scars, that form on neurons. MS results from progressive damage to the myelin sheathing that insulates and protects the neuron's axons. For reasons that remain a mystery, the immune systems of people who have MS attempt to destroy the body's own myelin. Specifically, a type of white blood cell called a T-cell becomes sensitized against myelin and eventually the myelin can be stripped away, damaging the supportive cells and eventually incapacitating or destroying the axon.[114]

Exposure to chemical toxins, such as organic solvents and pesticides, has been suggested as an MS trigger. Similarly, exposure to heavy metals, such as mercury, has also been implicated in MS. Mercury is widely known to affect neurological tissue.[115]

---

[112] Walton, J.R. (2007b) Human Range Dietary Aluminum Equivalents Cause Cognitive Deterioration in Aged Rats, (presented at the 24th International Neurotoxicology Conference, San Antonio, Texas, November, 2007)

[113] Noonan, C. W., Sarasua, S. M., Campagna, D., Kathman, S. J., Lybarger, J. A. & Mueller, P. W. (2002) Effects of exposure to low levels of environmental cadmium on renal biomarkers. *Environ Health Perspect 2002*(110), 151-155.

[114] Kidd, P. M. (2001) Multiple sclerosis, autoimmune inflammatory disease: prospects for its integrative management. *Alternative Medicine Review, 6*(6), 540-566.

[115] Mutter, J., Naumann, J. & Guethlin, C. (2007) Comments on the article the toxicology of mercury and its chemical compounds by Clarkson & Magos (2006) Crit. Rev. Toxicol., *37*, 537-549.Nadel, L. & Jacobs, W. J. 1998. Traumatic memory is special. *Curr. Dir.Psychol. Sci.* 7, 154–157.

## AUTOIMMUNE DISEASE

In the mid-1990s, Swedish researchers evaluated 13 studies on the connection between solvent exposure and autoimmune disease. Organic solvents were investigated such as toluene, paint thinner, and acetone, the last commonly found in nail polish remover. Ten of those studies indicated a significant relationship between organic solvent exposure and MS. All the analyses suggested that exposure to solvents increases a person's relative risk of developing MS.[116]

### THE HEALTH RISK FOR CHILDREN

Children are much more vulnerable to these toxins than adults. In March of 2003, the Environmental Protection Agency (EPA) reported that children run a much higher risk of developing cancer when exposed to mutagenic contaminants compared to adults. (Mutagenic contaminants are defined as "those agents that cause a permanent genetic change in a cell other than that which occurs during normal growth."[117])

For a child under the age of two, the EPA reported the risk at 10 times higher than adults, and for children aged two to15 it was increased two to five times. The key to this increase is that children are growing faster

---

[116] Landtblom, A.M., Tondel, M., Hjalmarsson, P., Flodin, U. & Axelson, O. (2005) The risk for multiple sclerosis in female nurse anaesthetists: a register based study. *Occup. Environ. Med.2006*(63), 387-389. doi:10.1136/oem.2005.024604

[117] U.S. Environmental Protection Agency (2003) Draft Final Guidelines for Carcinogen Risk Assessment (External Review Draft, February 2003). U.S. Environmental Protection Agency, Risk Assessment Forum, Washington, DC, 2003.

and their cells are dividing more rapidly, making their cells more vulnerable to DNA damage.

Doris Rapp, M.D. (H), author of *Our Toxic World*, researched the dangers we are facing with chemical pollutants we have dumped into our air, water, soil, food, homes, schools and workplace. Dr. Rapp lists the potential effects of these toxins on bodily systems:

- Our immune system: causes infections, allergies and cancer;
- Our endocrine system: causes thyroid, and adrenal disease, and diabetes;
- Our nervous system: causes learning and behavior problems;
- Our reproductive system: causes major sexual difficulties and changes.

Her research also suggests that ADHD, brain defects, and muscle and visual problems as well as many more issues are all related to this exposure.[118]

The impact of these toxins can be seen in the rising occurrence of disease in this country. For example, according to The Center for Disease Control, the Autism Spectrum Disorder (ASD) prevalence rate was 2 to 6 per 1,000 in 2001. We now see ASD in 1 out of every *88* births.[119]

---

[118] Rapp, D. (2003) *Our Toxic World: A Wake Up Call*. Raleigh, North Carolina: Environmental Research Foundation.
[119] Center for Disease Control (2009) Prevalence of Autism Spectrum Disorders-Autism and Developmental Disabilities Monitoring Network, United States, 2006. *Morbidity and Mortality Weekly Report, 2009* (58), SS-10.

In this chapter, we have only touched on a small fraction of the toxic exposures with which we come in contact every day. As our brains are affected by everything we drink, eat and breathe, it is essential for our future health that we all become aware of what is in our food, water and air. We cannot attempt to correct brain issues without examining what we can eliminate from our own environment that might otherwise be harmful to our families and ourselves.

## ENVIRONMENTAL HEALTH RISKS FOR ATHLETES

We think of athletes as virtually immune to the frailties of the typical human condition. They are, after all, perfect examples of physical prowess: a very healthy lifestyle, lots of exercise, and a healthy diet. But some health risks actually strike *more* athletes than their less athletic peers.

As an athlete, minimizing exposure to toxins in the environment is crucial. Because an athlete plays harder and longer than most, s/he has a much higher chance of coming and staying in contact with toxic environments than non-athletes. These toxins can cause neurological damage and other diseases such as cancer, Parkinson's disease, Alzheimer's disease and ALS.

### CARDIOVASCULAR DISEASE

Cardiovascular disease seems to be rising in young athletes. In September, 2005 the deaths of 14 young athletes were reported in a Southern California newspaper in the article entitled "Heart of the

Matter." [120] Ten of the 14 deaths were male athletes who were under 21 years of age. The youngest was just 13!

Sudden cardiac arrest caused by *hypertrophic cardiomyopathy* (HCM) is often to blame. HCM is an inherited condition which causes the heart's main pumping chamber, the left ventricle, to be abnormally thick.

In 1966, the Journal of the American Medical Association (JAMA) published a study of 158 sudden deaths that had occurred in trained athletes throughout the United States between 1985 and 1995.[121] The athletes were all young—high school and college-aged athletes. Of those 158 athletes, 134 suffered from cardiovascular causes of sudden death and the most common cause was HCM.

Other causes of sudden cardiac death in this study included myocarditis, an inflammation of the heart muscle, and coronary artery abnormalities. Researchers reported that approximately 90% of these athletes collapsed during or immediately after a training session. They theorized that physical exertion appeared to trigger sudden death.

---

[120] Smith, M.C. Heart of the matter. *The Orange County Register*, p-11, 9-25-05.
[121] Maron BJ, Thompson PD, Puffer JC, et al. Cardiovascular pre-participation screening of competitive athletes. A statement for health professionals from the Sudden Death Committee (clinical cardiology) and Congenital Cardiac Defects Committee (cardiovascular disease in the young), American Heart Association. *Circulation* . 1996;15;94(4):850-6.

The current recommendation from the American Heart Association is to screen all athletes for heart irregularities. Since there is a large cost associated with screening every athlete and because approximately 6% of the screenings come back as false positives, athletic teams and schools are looking at installing CPR machines in case of a cardiac failure incident.[122]

Unfortunately, these recommendations will do little to stop the emerging epidemic of cardiovascular disease and premature death among serious athletes. The reasons for this are the lack of attention to the nutritional health and the health-negative effects of other factors affecting athletes such as:

1.  Nutrient deficient foods that contain chemical additives.
2.  Environmental toxins found in our food supply, water and air.
3.  Electromagnetic pollution.
4.  Stress damage caused by excessive exercise.
5.  Overuse of prescription drugs for treating all health and injury related issues.

## ATHLETE'S HEART

Another issue common to athletes is *athlete's heart*.[123] This usually occurs in athletes who train more than an hour a day. Athlete's heart (or *athletic brachycardia*), occurs when the volume and pressure loads in the

---

[122] American Heart Association (2009, July 29). Proper Placement Of Defibrillators Key To Effective Use. *ScienceDaily*. Retrieved from http://www.sciencedaily.com/releases/2009/07/090727191904.htm
[123] Lohr, J. T. (1999) *Athletic Heart Syndrome*. Gale Encyclopedia of Medicine.

heart's left ventricle (LV) increase. Over time, this will increase the LV muscle mass, wall thickness, and chamber size. The result is that the heart beats unusually slowly, typically under 60 beats per minute. Although this condition is believed to be benign, it may be hard to distinguish from other serious medical conditions.

## AMYOTROPHIC LATERAL SCLEROSIS (ALS) OR LOU GEHRIG'S DISEASE

Amyotrophic lateral sclerosis (ALS) or Lou Gehrig's disease is a form of motor neuron disease. ALS is caused by the degeneration of motor neurons, the nerve cells in the central nervous system that control voluntary muscle movement. In the US, this condition is often referred to as Lou Gehrig's disease, after the famous New York Yankees baseball player who was diagnosed with the disease in 1939. The disorder causes muscle weakness and atrophy throughout the body.[124]

According to a 2002 Columbia University study, people who develop motor neuron afflictions, including ALS, are more likely to be lean of build and to have been varsity athletes.[125]

---

[124] Beal, M.F., Lang, A.E. & Ludolph, A.C. (2005) *Neurodegenerative Diseases: Neurobiology, Pathogenesis and Therapeutics*. Cambridge: Cambridge University Press. p. 775. ISBN 0-521-81166-X. OCLC 57691713

[125] N. Scarmeas, MD; T. Shih, MD; Y. Stern, PhD; R. Ottman, PhD; and L.P. Rowland, MD (2002) Premorbid weight, body mass, and varsity athletics in ALS. *Neurology* 2002;59:773–775

The study compared characteristics of 229 people who had developed muscle nerve degeneration with 152 others having other types of neurological diseases. Body mass index (BMI), gender, age and participation in varsity athletics were considered. According to Dr. Nikolaos Scarmeas, lead author of the study, "The odds of having motor neuron disease was 2.21 times higher in subjects who reported they had always been slim than in those who did not. Further, motor neuron disease was 1.70 times higher in patients who reported they had been varsity athletes." [126]

The study also offered an explanation of the association with nerve diseases and athletes. Researchers theorized that vigorous physical activity might increase exposure to environmental toxins that can damage nerves or that activity might make it easier for those toxins to reach the brain or increase their absorption.

Cardiovascular disease and diseases like ALS are not the only things that affect athletes.

*MARATHON RUNNERS*

Over the years, several marathon runners have died in unusual circumstances. Most had pre-existing heart conditions, but not all. On December 14, 2008, a veteran distance runner collapsed during the White Rock Marathon in Dallas, Texas and later died in the hospital. There was no immediate determination of the cause of her collapse.

---

[126] N. Scarmeas, MD; T. Shih, MD; Y. Stern, PhD; R. Ottman, PhD; and L.P. Rowland, MD (2002) Premorbid weight, body mass, and varsity athletics in ALS. NEUROLOGY 2002;59:773–775

Another cause has been identified as *hyponatremia*, an abnormally low sodium level in the blood. This can be caused by drinking only water and not replacing electrolytes lost while running. Heat exhaustion and heat stroke have also caused runners to be sent to the hospital after even a short distance event. Endurance athletes put themselves at even higher risk although deaths among marathon runners are still relatively rare. A study by Dr. Bill Roberts, the medical director of the Twin Cities Marathon, showed the risk of dying from a heart attack in a marathon is about one in 75,000 finishers. Compare this to the annual risk of dying in a car accident at 1:6,535[127]

## TOXIC ENVIRONMENTS AND ATHLETES

Athletes are exposed to specific kinds of toxins in their environments that are not typically in the environments of those of us who are not athletes.

### SYNTHETIC TURF

Natural grass fields in sports complexes are increasingly being replaced with artificial (or synthetic) turf. These new generation fields are designed to mimic the look and feel of natural grass and are hailed as more cost-effective and durable. From the beginning with the 1967 *AstroTurf*, created by the Ford Foundation and Monsanto. Today more than 3,500 artificial turf fields are currently in use

---

[127] Capozzi, J. (2008) Marathons safe if you train, risky if you don't. Retrieved from http://www.palmbeachpost.com/sports/content/sports/epaper/2008/12/04/1204marathon.html

across North America with an additional 1,000 fields being installed every year.

This first generation of synthetic turf was essentially a short pile carpet with a foam backing. Since then, design changes have resulted in a greater variety of synthetic turf athletic fields. The turf is created in multiple layers to mimic the look and feel of real grass. The artificial 'grass blades' are made of recycled plastics and polymers that include polyethylene, polypropylene and nylon.[128]

Surfaces are filled with bits of recycled tires (called crumb rubber) to provide a cushioned platform. These tire bits are usually less than 3 millimeters in diameter and are manufactured from natural and synthetic rubbers along with numerous chemical additives, including zinc, sulfur, carbon black, and oils that contain polyaromatic hydrocarbons (PAHs) and volatile organic chemicals. Because crumb rubber is manufactured from used tires, it probably contains the same chemicals as tire rubber.

Synthetic turf is typically divided into two types, one with fill material in between the blades of "grass" and the others without. There is growing concern that those that use fill are contaminated with toxic chemicals—including PAHs and metals—in the artificial grass blades or in the surface. The substances, which may end up in the air, on skin or in mouths, can

---

[128] Daines, R.F. & Saunders, W.E. (2008) *FACT SHEET:Crumb-Rubber Infilled Synthetic Turf Athletic Fields, August 2008.* State of New York Department of Health.

pose a health risk through breathing or eating for children, athletes and others who use the fields. [129]

## HEALTH AND SAFETY CONSIDERATIONS

It is generally agreed that injuries are more likely on a synthetic turf field. Heat has been found to be an issue as well. The surface temperature of an artificial turf field can be much higher than the air temperature. Artificial field surface temperatures have been documented as high as 199°F on a sunny day with an air temperature of 98°F. Researchers at Brigham Young University reported that the surface temperature of a synthetic football field on campus averaged 117°F, with a daily high of 157°F. [130] On an adjacent natural grass field the surface temperature averaged 78°F, with a daily high of 89°F.

Researchers at Penn State University studied the effect of using irrigation to reduce surface temperatures of synthetic fields and discovered that temperature could be decreased with irrigation, but the effects were short-lived, on the order of 20 minutes. [131] Because of these high temperatures, an artificial field will remain largely unusable during warm days. Additionally,

---

[129] Brakeman, L. (2004) Infill systems spark debate at STMA conference. Retrieved from:
http://www.athleticturf.net/athleticturf/content/printContentPopup.jsp?id=85955 .
[130] Williams C.F., & G.E. Pulley. (2003) Synthetic surface heat studies. Available at:
http://cahe.nmsu.edu/programs/turf/documents/brigham-young-study.pdf .
[131] McNitt, A.S., D.M. Petrunak, & T.J. Serensits. (2008) Temperature amelioration of synthetic turf surfaces through irrigation. Acta Hort. 783:573-581, ISHS 2008.

practicing on an artificial field could increase the incidence of heat stroke, muscle cramping, and overall athlete fatigue.

## INFECTION RISK

An aspect of synthetic turf that is now receiving increased scrutiny is the potential for increased incidences of infections among players that play primarily on in-fill systems. In a report entitled "Texas Football Succumbs to Virulent Staph Infection from Turf", at least 276 football players were reported to be infected with an antibiotic-resistant staph infection (MRSA), a rate of 517 for each 100,000 individuals. [132] The U.S. Centers for Disease Control and Prevention in Atlanta reported a rate for the general population of 32 in 100,000.

These infections were primarily associated with increased skin abrasions associated with synthetic turf and the risk of infection that might occur off the field from infections.

In-fill systems must now be routinely treated with special disinfectants to reduce the likelihood of infections, adding yet another layer of toxins to these fields.

---

[132] Epstein, V. (2007) Texas football succumbs to virulent staph infection from turf. Retrieved from: http://www.bloomberg.com/apps/news?pid=20601109&sid=alxhrJDn. cdc&refer=news; Data compiled from the Texas Department of State Health Services, http://www.dshs.state.tx.us/idcu/health/antibiotic_resistanc e/mrsa/

## HEAVY METALS EXPOSURE

Lead has been known for centuries to be toxic to humans. Yet it wasn't until the 1970s that lead was banned from paints and gasoline. Lead was even used in the manufacture of water pipes. Today there are much more stringent restrictions and the general population is much more aware of the dangers of lead exposure.

Despite this new found awareness, in April 2008, New Jersey officials found elevated lead levels in artificial turf playing fields.[133] Some types of synthetic turf fibers contain elevated levels of lead (e.g., in the range of about 2,000 to 9,000 parts per million). Degradation of these fibers can form a dust that presents a potential source of lead exposure to users of the fields. The Centers for Disease Control and Prevention and the Agency for Toxic Substances and Disease Registry addressed the potential for lead exposure from synthetic turf fibers in a June 2008 Health Advisory. [134]

## AIR POLLUTANTS FOR COMPETITION

Air pollution is an oft-ignored issue for athletes. According to Dr. Kenneth Rundell, the director of the Human Performance Laboratory at Marywood University in Scranton, Pennsylvania, "Athletes typically take in 10 to 20 times as much air, and thus 10 to 20 times the pollutants, with every breath as

---

[133] McCarthy, M. & Berkowitz, S. (2008) Artificial Turf: Health Hazard? *USA Today* (may 7,2008)
[134] Center for Disease Control (2010) Artificial Turf. Retrieved from http://www.cdc.gov/nceh/lead/tips/artificialturf.htm

sedentary people do." Although experts continue to say people should not stop exercising outside, they caution exercisers to keep their distance from cars emitting heavy exhaust fumes and check air-quality before starting their exercise routines.

A 2004 review of pollution studies worldwide conducted by the University of Brisbane, Australia, found that during exercise, low concentrations of pollutants caused lung damage similar to that caused by high concentrations in people not working out.[135] Therefore, the long-term consequences of pollution exposure for athletes might be much more harmful than their more sedentary counterparts.

Although according to Dr. Michelle Bell, an assistant professor of environmental health at the Yale School of Forestry and Environmental Studies, "...[o]zone over the long term causes what is similar to a premature aging of the lungs", today most experts agree that the greatest overall public health impact of air pollution comes from fine particulates which can be seen only with an electron microscope.

These tiny particles are pervasive in our environment coming from an ever-increasing supply of cars, trucks and diesel buses—the main culprits in the creation of particle pollution. They spew millions of these microscopic pollutants into our air daily. Particles can sail past nasal hairs, the body's first line of defense, and settle deep in the lungs. Some remain there, causing

---

[135] Hansen,C.A., Barnett,A.G., Jalaludin, B.B. & Morgan, G.G. (2004) Ambient Air Pollution and Birth Defects in Brisbane, Australia. PLoS ONE 4(4): e5408. doi:10.1371/journal.pone.0005408

irritation and inflammation. Others, so tiny they can bypass various bodily defenses, migrate into the bloodstream.

Air pollution is also a known trigger for asthma and the type of particulate matter commonly found in urban air can sometimes lead to more severe asthma attacks, hospitalization or death. Athletes with asthma are particularly vulnerable. [136] They will experience a greater decrease in their lung function if the smog rolls in.

Further, a study included in the Women's Health Initiative found that women who lived in communities with relatively high levels of air pollution in the forms of tiny particles—also known as soot—were far more likely to die because of heart attacks than women who lived in cleaner air.[137]

Another primary concern to athletes should be carbon monoxide. This is a gas that can kill you if you're locked in a room with a running automobile, but because it's clear, odorless, and doesn't cause smog, it has largely drifted below the media radar.

Usually athletes won't experience any long-term damage from carbon monoxide, but "...for competition,

---

[136] Archer,A.J., Cramton, J.L., Pfau, J.P., Colasurdo,G. & Holian, A. (2003) Airway responsiveness after acute exposure to urban particulate matter. Am J Physiol Lung Cell Mol Physiol 286: L337-L343, 2004.

[137] Miller, K.A., Siscovick, D.S., Sheppard, L., Shepherd, K., Sullivan, J.H., Anderson, G.L. et al (2007) Long-Term Exposure to Air Pollution and Incidence of Cardiovascular Events in Women. *N Engl J Med* 2007; 356:447-458February 1, 2007

this is a serious concern," says Philip S. Clifford, who researches respiratory function at the Medical College of Wisconsin. Studies of athletes exercising close to heavy traffic have shown carbon monoxide levels of about 5 percent in the blood—similar to the level in a smoker who just indulged—meaning that the capacity to carry oxygen in the blood to the body has been reduced 5 percent. "That could really make an impact on aerobic performance," Clifford says. "And the impact might not be spread out equally."

Clifford theorizes that athletes who have a lower hematocrit (that proportion of blood that is oxygen-carrying red blood cells) will feel the effects more acutely than their high-hematocrit counterparts. Because women generally have lower levels of hemoglobin and fewer red blood cells than men, if Clifford's suggestion is correct, female athletes may be more affected by carbon monoxide.

The bottom line is that, even if you're not a runner or elite endurance athlete, listen to your body. As your brain is affected by everything you drink, eat and breathe, it is essential for your future health that you become aware of what is in your food, water and air. You can't correct brain issues without first examining what you can eliminate from your own environment that might be harmful to yourself and your family.

# CHAPTER 6
# MEDICATING
# THE BRAIN

Science has made great advances in medicine that have helped us live longer lives and overcome horrendous ills and infections of the past. Vaccines to eliminate diseases such as polio and smallpox have been developed as well as others to improve the outcomes of diseases such as rabies, diphtheria and the plague.

However, because of our longer life spans, the processed foods we eat, the fast-paced lives we live and the chemicals that pollute our world, we are facing a host of new health problems. Solutions have typically focused on medications to alleviate symptoms rather than simpler, more basic—and potentially more effective—changes, such as diet, exercise and lifestyle.

Pharmaceutical companies have saturated our airways with advertisements that make prescription drugs seem like the only answer. Smiling people tell us how the next great drug will improve our lives. Following the pitch, however, is the mandated and often lengthy list of potential side effects, recited quickly in a much lower tone of voice with a relaxing and cheerful musical background. "Anal leakage?" "Potentially fatal?" Some cures may just be worse than the diseases.

# NEUROTRANSMITTERS

Neurotransmitters are substances produced in our bodies and brains and used by the nervous system to control body functions and emotions. They are typically manufactured in the nerve cell body and then transported to its terminal end. When there is a signal—an Action Potential—that stimulates a transmitting neuron, the neurotransmitter is released from the terminal area and moves across the gap, or *synapse*, to the next, the receiving neuron. Some neurotransmitters such as norepinephrine, dopamine and serotonin, may be reabsorbed into the terminal region of the originating neuron. This phenomenon is called "reuptake."

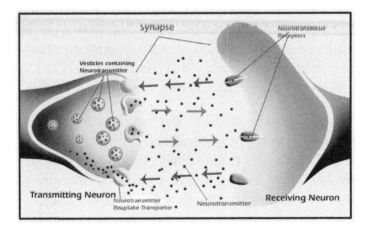

**Fig. 6-1**

At the other side of the synapse, neurotransmitters encounter receptors. A neurotransmitter binds only to a specific type or types of receptors, similar to the way in which a key fits into a lock. This key-like selectivity prevents all neurotransmitters from binding to all receptors. To further complicate matters, some neurotransmitters have different effects depending upon the receptor to which they bind. For example, acetylcholine can be stimulatory when bound to one receptor and inhibitory when bound to another.

When a receptor site recognizes a neurotransmitter, it is activated. This can result in an alternative mechanism, stimulating or inhibiting the release of the neurotransmitter. Thus we have a means of control over how quickly and when information can pass from neuron to neuron. The binding of a neurotransmitter to a receptor triggers a biological effect.

Once the process is complete, however, its ability to stimulate the biological effect is lost. The receptor then must bind another neurotransmitter molecule in order to repeat the stimulating effect.

Here is a partial list of known neurotransmitters:

- **Acetylcholine**: Acetylcholine is particularly important in the stimulation of muscle tissue. After stimulation, acetylcholine degrades to acetate and choline, which are absorbed back into the first neuron to form another acetylcholine molecule.[138] However, the poison curare blocks transmission of acetylcholine and some nerve gases and most chlorinated hydrocarbon insecticides (quite similar to the structure of the artificial sweetener

---

[138] Philp, R.B. (2013) *Ecosystems and Human Health: 2ⁿᵈ Edition*. LEWIS PUBLISHERS:Boca Raton London New York Washington, D.C.

Splenda®) inhibit the breakdown of acetylcholine, producing a continuous stimulation of the receptor cells, and spasms of muscles such as the heart.[139]

- **Epinephrine (adrenaline) and norepinephrine:** These compounds are secreted mainly by the adrenal gland. Secretion causes an increased heart rate and the enhanced production of glucose as a ready energy source (the "fight or flight" response).[140]

- **Dopamine:** Dopamine facilitates critical brain functions and, when unusual quantities are present, abnormal dopamine neurotransmission may play a role in Parkinson's disease, certain addictions, and schizophrenia.[141]

- **Serotonin:** Synthesized from the amino acid tryptophan, serotonin is assumed to play a biochemical role in mood and mood disorders, including anxiety, depression, and bipolar disorder.[142]

- **Aspartate:** An amino acid that stimulates neurons in the central nervous system,

---

[139] Jurewicz, J.& Hanke, W. (9 Jul 2008) Prenatal and Childhood Exposure to Pesticides and Neurobehavioral Development: Review of Epidemiological Studies. *International Journal of Occupational Medicine and Environmental Health* (Versita, Warsaw) 21 (2): 121–132.
[140] von Bohlen und Halbach, O & Dermietzel, R (2006) *Neurotransmitters and neuromodulators: handbook of receptors and biological effects.* Wiley-VCH. p. 125.
[141] Björklund A, Dunnett SB (May 2007) Dopamine neuron systems in the brain: an update. *Trends Neurosci.* 30 (5): 194–202.
[142] Young SN (2007) How to increase serotonin in the human brain without drugs. *Rev. Psychiatr. Neurosci.* 32 (6): 394–99.

particularly those that transfer information to the area of the brain called the cerebrum. Aspartate is a breakdown product of the artificial sweetener Aspartame®.[143]

- **Oxytocin:** A short protein (peptide) that is released within the brain, ovary, and testes. The compound stimulates the release of milk by mammary glands, contractions during birth, and maternal behavior.[144]
- **Somatostatin:** Another peptide which is inhibitory to the secretion of growth hormone from the pituitary gland, of insulin, and of a variety of gastrointestinal hormones involved with nutrient absorption.[145]
- **Insulin:** A peptide secreted by the pancreas that stimulates other cells to absorb glucose.[146]

As you can see, each neurotransmitter acts uniquely. However, their effects may change as well, depending upon the receptors to which they bind.

[143] Lehninger, Albert L.; Nelson, David L.; Cox, Michael M. (2000), *Principles of Biochemistry* (3rd ed.), New York: W. H. Freeman,
[144] Lee, H.J., Macbeth, A.H., Pagani, J.H. & Young, W.S. (June 2009) Oxytocin: the great facilitator of life. *Prog. Neurobiol.* 88 (2): 127–51.
[145] Costoff, A. (2008) Sect. 5, Ch. 4: Structure, Synthesis, and Secretion of Somatostatin. *Endocrinology: The Endocrine Pancreas*. Medical College of Georgia. pp. page 16.
[146] Benedict C, Hallschmid M, Hatke A, Schultes B, Fehm HL, Born J, Kern W. (November 2004) Intranasal insulin improves memory in humans. *Psychoneuroendocrinology* 29 (10): 1326–34.

# ADHD

Attention Deficit Hyperactivity Disorder (ADHD) has become a national epidemic. The term has been redefined as an umbrella diagnosis in the Diagnostic and Statistical Manual of Mental Disorders, Fourth Edition (DSM-IV) and includes all forms of attention deficit, including those called predominantly inattentive, predominantly hyperactive and combined.

The number of children in America diagnosed with ADHD is growing each year. According to the CDC and The National Health Institutes, 5-8% of children ages 3-17 (4.7 million) are currently diagnosed with ADHD. Twice as many boys as girls are affected between the ages of six and 17.

The US has only 2% of the world's population, but we consume more than 85% of the Ritalin manufactured in the world.[147]

At one point in 2006, 9.6 million children in the United States had been taking prescribed ADHD medications for at least four consecutive months.[148]

Studies have shown that these drugs are only a short-term fix, *if* they work at all. The eight-year follow-up data from the ADHD MTA (Multisite Multimodal

---

[147] Montandon, J. B., & Medioni, L. (2001) Evolution of the number of prescriptions of Ritalin (Methylphenidate) in the Canton of Neuchatel between 1996-2000, *Pharmaceutical Control and Authorization Division, Switzerland.*

[148] Center for Disease Control (2006) Summary Health Statistics for U.S. Children: National Health Interview Survey, 2006. Retrieved from: *www.cdc.gov/nchs/data/series/sr_10/sr10_234.pdf*

Treatment Study of Children with Attention Deficit/Hyperactivity Disorder) suggests that use of ADHD drugs for more than two years is ineffective.

Not only are symptomatic benefits reduced with chronic use of these medications, the latest study also suggests that long-term use of medication may also impair growth. The study found children who took ADHD medication for 36 months or longer were, on average, six pounds lighter and one inch shorter than their peers.[149,150]

Even more disturbing than the prescription of ADHD medications to school-age children is the trend to prescribing this medication to *preschool* children aged one to three years. As you will recall from Chapter 2, these small children are still "living" in their limbic brains. They are just beginning to learn how to control their emotions with their immature prefrontal cortices. Issues with reasoning, emotions and problem-solving are common and appropriate at this age. The frontal lobes that are so crucial in reasoning, planning,

---

[149] Molina, B. S. G., Hinshaw, S. P., Swanson, J. M., Arnold, L. E., Vitiello, B., Jensen, P.S., et al. (2006) The MTA at 8 years: Prospective follow-up of children treated for combined type ADHD in the multisite study. *Journal of the American Academy of Child and Adolescent Psychiatry.* Retrieved from: http://www.nimh.nih.gov/science-news/2009/shortterm-intensive-treatment-not-likely-to-improve-long-term-outcomes-for-children-withADHD.shtml

[150] Jensen, P. S., et al. (2007) 3-year follow-up of the NIMH MTA Study. *Journal of the American Academy of Child and Adolescent Psychiatry, 46* (8), 989–1002.

movement, emotions, and problem solving simply do not mature until 20 years of age or older. [151]

Since the most common such medication, methylphenidate (Ritalin®), works primarily in the prefrontal cortex[152], it seems to make little sense to prescribe it in infants and preschoolers. In addition, children are no longer just taking the medicines for a few years during grade school but are encouraged to stay on them into adulthood. In 2008, two stimulants—Vyvanse® (lisdexamfetamine) and Concerta® (another brand of time-release methylphenidate)—received U.S. Food and Drug Administration approval for treating adults. Thus, pharmaceutical firms are now allowed to advertise these medications to adults for their own use.

In addition to all those who are diagnosed with ADHD, we are now seeing "off label" use by people who have no cognitive deficits, but who choose to take these drugs in hopes of boosting academic or business performance. As a result, prescriptions for methylphenidate and amphetamine rose by almost 12 percent a year between 2000 and 2005.[153]

Concern is mounting that the drugs might take a greater toll on the brain over the long run than was

---

[151] Cauffman, E. et. al. (2010) Age Differences in Affective Decision Making as Indexed by Performance on the Iowa Gambling Test , *DEV. PSYCHOL. 46* (193).

[152] Devilbiss, M. & Berridge, C. W. (2008) Cognition-Enhancing Doses of Methylphenidate Preferentially Increase Prefrontal Cortex Neuronal Responsiveness. *Biological Psychiatry, 64* (7), 626-635.

[153] Watkins, C.E. (2006) New Medications for Adults with ADHD. Retrieved from: http://www.ncpamd.com/NewADD_Meds.htm

first anticipated. A team led by psychologist Stacy A. Castner of the Yale University School of Medicine documented hallucinations and cognitive impairment in Rhesus monkeys that received escalating injections of amphetamines over 6-12 weeks.[154]

In 2005, The University of Texas M.D. Anderson Cancer Center completed a study using Ritalin to relieve symptoms of ADHD. In this study, 12 children were given standard therapeutic doses of methylphenidate. At the conclusion of the three-month study, all 12 children displayed significant, treatment-induced chromosomal aberrations, indicating that methylphenidate is almost certainly carcinogenic.[155]

Other studies have shown that Ritalin use in children increases chances of drug abuse and developing chronic drug dependency in adolescence,[156] and causes permanent brain damage in both animals[157] and

---

[154] Castner, S., Vosler, P. & Goldman-Rakic, P.S. (2005) Amphetamine sensitization impairs cognition and reduces dopamine turnover in primate prefrontal cortex. *Biological Psychiatry. 57* (7), 743-751. doi:10.1016/j.biopsych.2004.12.019

[155] El-Zein, R. A., Abdel-Rahman, S. Z., Hay, M.J., Lopez, M. S., Bondy, M. L., Morris, D. L., et al. (2005) *Cytogenetic effects in children treated with methylphenidate. Department of Epidemiology*, Houston, TX: The University of Texas M.D. Anderson Cancer Center, PMID: 16297714

[156] Mannuzza, S., Klein, R. G. , Truong, N. L., Moulton III, J. L. , Roizen, E. R. , Howell, K. H. et al.(2008) Age of Methylphenidate Treatment Initiation in Children With ADHD and Later Substance Abuse: Prospective Follow-Up Into Adulthood. *Am J Psychiatry, 165*(5), 604 – 609.

[157] Kuroda, N. (2000) Effects of *Metilphenidate* on brain function in mice. *Tokyo Veterinary. Society Bulletin, 128*, 36-62.

---

humans.[158] Ritalin has been conclusively shown to be the leading cause of increasing rates of drug-induced schizophrenia, depression, and bipolar disorder in children in North America. [159],[160],[161]

Use of Ritalin in the USA still continues to increase. The fact that a large proportion of American children are being routinely medicated with a drug that is potentially highly destructive raises serious questions in this writer's mind about the relationship among the pharmaceutical industry, the FDA, health insurers, and health care providers.

## ADHD MEDICATIONS

Until recently, scientists believed that the cause of ADHD was low levels of dopamine. However, new evidence suggests it is not just the level of dopamine that is an issue, but higher than normal levels of

---

[158] Breggin, P.R. (1990) Brain Damage, Dementia and Persistent Cognitive Dysfunction Associated with Neuroleptic Drugs: Evidence, Etiology, Implications. *Journal of Mind Behavior, 11*, 425-464.

[159] Breggin, P. R. (1999) Psychostimulants in the treatment of children diagnosed with ADHD: Part I — Acute risks and psychological effects. *Ethical Human Sciences and Services, 1*, 23-28. Available from Sage publications database.

[160] Cherland, E., & Fitzpatrick, R. (1999) Psychotic Side Effects of Psychostimulants: A 5-year review. *Canadian Journal of Psychiatry, 44*, 811-813. Retrieved from: http://www.drakeinstitute.com/research-article/psychotic-side-effects.pdf

[161] Gillberg, C., Melander, H., von Knorring, A-L., Janols, L-O., Thernlund, G., Hagglof, B., et al. (1997) Long-term stimulant treatment of children with attention-deficit hyperactivity disorder symptoms: A randomized, double-blind, placebo-controlled trial. *Archives of General Psychiatry 54*, 857-864.

dopamine *transporters* in the part of the brain called the striatum that helps us plan ahead.[162],[163]

Transporters are those chemicals that move the dopamine across the synapse to the receiving neuron and then allow part of the dopamine to be reabsorbed into the sending neuron, the so-called reuptake mechanism. People with ADHD appear to have an overabundance of these transporters, as compared to the number of receptors. The result is that the dopamine does not have sufficient time to exert its effects before it is reabsorbed.

The majority of patients on ADHD medications are prescribed either methylphenidate (Ritalin, Concerta) or an amphetamine (Adderall, Vyvanse). Medications such as Ritalin block the dopamine transporters and prevent reuptake of the dopamine after it's released, resulting in an excess of dopamine.

Dopamine syndrome occurs when the body has a high excess of dopamine from extended or overuse of these dopamine-reuptake inhibitors. The effects produced by excessive dopamine in the system are:

---

[162] Browman, K.E., Curzon, P., Pan, J. B., Molesky, A. L., Komater, V.A., Decker, M. W. et al. (2005) GB. A-412997, a selective dopamine D4 agonist, improves cognitive performance in rats. *Pharmacology, Biochemistry and Behaviour. 82* (1), 148-55. PMID 16154186
[163] Heijtz, R. D., Kolb, B. & Forssberg, H. (2007) Motor inhibitory role of dopamine D1 receptors: implications for ADHD. *Physiol Behav ,92* (1-2), 155–160. doi:10.1016/j.physbeh.2007.05.024. PMID 17585966. Retrieved from:
http://www.sciencedirect.com/science?_ob=MImg&_imagekey=B6T0P-4NTB97R-Y1&_cdi=4868&_user=308069&_orig=search&_coverDate=09%2F30%2F2007&_sk=999079998&view=c&wchp=dGLbVzz-zSkzV&md5=c49d721e7e713190 c2ac6fab7a491093&ie=/sdarticle.pdf.

## PSYCHOLOGICAL

- Disorientation and/or confusion
- Anxiety, severe paranoia, and/or panic attacks
- Hyper-vigilance or increased sensitivity to perceptual stimuli, accompanied by significantly increased threat detection
- Hypomania or full-blown mania
- De-realization and/or depersonalization (being disconnected to the world or oneself)
- Hallucinations and/or delusions
- Thought disorder or disorganized thinking
- Cognitive and memory impairment potentially to the point of retrograde or anterograde amnesia
- Delirium and/or insanity

## PHYSIOLOGICAL

- Myoclonus or involuntary and intense muscle twitching
- Hyperreflexia or over-responsive/over-reactive reflexes

Miscellaneous

- Syncope or fainting including loss of consciousness
- Seizures or convulsions
- Neurotoxicity or brain damage
- Coma and/or death

Although there have been no clinical studies performed on the long-term effects on the brains of adults or children who use safe doses of Ritalin, there have been many studies on the effects of long-term stimulant abuse on the brain. The long-term use of any drug that affects the brain's reward circuitry also raises the possibility of addiction.

Ritalin has a chemical structure similar to that of cocaine and acts on the brain in a very similar way. Both cocaine and methamphetamine, another highly addictive stimulant, block dopamine transporters—just as ADHD drugs do.[164] In the case of the illicit drugs, the dopamine surge is so sudden that in addition to making a person unusually energetic and alert, it produces a "high."[165]

In February 2009, neuroscientists Yong Kim and Paul Greengard, along with their colleagues at the Rockefeller University, reported cocaine-like structural and chemical alterations in the brains of mice given methylphenidate.[166] They also found that methylphenidate boosted a protein called FosB, which turns genes on and off, even more than cocaine. That result could be a warning of future problems.

Many former cocaine addicts struggle with depression, anxiety and cognitive problems. Researchers have found that cocaine has remodeled the brains of such

---

[164] Sergo, P. (2008) New Weapons against Cocaine Addiction. *Scientific American Mind*, Retrieved from: http://www.scientificamerican.com/article.cfm?id=new-weapons-against-cocaine-addiction

[165] Brown, J.M., Hanson, G.R. & Fleckenstein, A.E. (2000) Methamphetamine Rapidly Decreases Vesicular Dopamine Uptake. *J Neurochem* 2000 May; 74(5):2221-3

[166] Horstman, J. (2010) *The Scientific American Brave New Brain.* Wiley: Hobokan, NJ.

ex-users. Similar problems—principally, perhaps, difficulty experiencing joy and excitement in life— could occur after years of Ritalin or Adderall use.[167]

## EFFECTS ON THE BODY

Addiction is not the only issue with drugs such as Ritalin. Long-term side effects from the abuse of Ritalin may also include loss of appetite that can lead to malnutrition, seizures, heart murmurs or cardiac arrest. Fevers, headaches, and the development of obsessive habits, such as nervous hand-wringing have also been noted.[168]

With the expanded and extended use of stimulants comes mounting concern that the drugs might take a toll on the brain over the long run. Indeed, recent studies, most of them involving animals, hint that stimulants could alter the structure and function of the brain in ways that may depress mood, boost anxiety and, contrary to their short-term effects, lead to cognitive deficits. Human studies already indicate that the medications can adversely affect areas of the brain that govern growth in children, as we saw with the Castner study earlier in this chapter.

In February 2006, the drug safety and risk committee of the Food and Drug Administration (FDA)

[167] Kim, Y., Teylan, M. A., Baron, M., Sands, A., Nairn, A. C., & Greengard, P. (2009) Methylphenidate-induced dendritic spine formation and ÄFosB expression in nucleus accumbens. *National Academy of Sciences Repository*. doi 10.1073/pnas.0813179106
[168] Hay, M. J., El-Zein, R. A., Lopez, M. S. , Bondy, M. L., & Morris, D. L. (2005) Chromosome damaging effect of small doses of Ritalin (Methylphenidate). *Cancer Letters. 230* ( 2), 284-291

recommended that all ADHD medications should carry a 'black box' warning of the risk of cardiac failure and sudden death, following a report listing 25 sudden deaths in both adults and children, between 1999 and 2003.

The following is a list of side effects that we know have occurred with methylphenidate (Ritalin) and dextroamphetamine (Dexadrine).

### *SIDE EFFECTS OF METHYLPHENIDATE* [169]

- Abdominal pain
- Feeling or being sick
- Dry mouth
- Fast heart rate
- Palpitations
- Irregular heart beat
- Changes in blood pressure
- Insomnia
- Nervousness
- Loss of appetite
- Headache
- Drowsiness
- Dizziness
- Movement disorders
- Painful joints
- Rashes, itching, hair loss
- Inflammation of blood vessels in the brain
- Angina (heart pain)

---

[169] King, S., Griffin, S., Hodges, Z., et al. (2006) A systematic review and economic model of the effectiveness and cost-effectiveness of methylphenidate, dexamfetamine and atomoxetine for the treatment of attention deficit hyperactivity disorder in children and adolescents. *Health Technol Assess* 10(23), iii–iv, xiii–146. PMID 16796929

- Hyperactivity
- Fits
- Psychosis (loss of contact with reality)
- Tics including Tourette's syndrome
- Neuroleptic malignant syndrome (a serious condition more commonly associated with antipsychotic drugs, involving high fever, tremor and rigidity and changes in consciousness)
- Drug dependence
- Growth retardation
- Reduced weight gain
- Blood disorders
- Muscle cramps
- Visual disturbances
- Peeling skin
- Erythema multiforme (raised red patches on the skin)

## SIDE EFFECTS OF DEXAMPHETAMINE [170] (DEXTROAMPHETAMINE)

- Sleeplessness
- Restlessness
- Irritability and excitability
- Nervousness
- Night terrors
- Euphoria
- Shaking
- Dizziness

---

[170] Efron, D., Jarman, F., Barker, M. (1997) Side effects of methylphenidate and dexamphetamine in children with attention deficit hyperactivity disorder: a double-blind, crossover trial.*Pediatrics. 100* (4), 662.

- Headache
- Fits
- Becoming dependent on the drug
- Sometimes psychosis
- Loss of appetite
- Gastro-intestinal symptoms
- Slowed growth in children
- Dry mouth
- Sweating
- Fast heart beat
- Palpitations
- Raised blood pressure
- Visual disturbances
- Heart muscle problems with long-term use
- Movement disorders
- Tics
- Tourette's syndrome

You should consider carefully whether to expose your child to stimulant drugs such as these; you may decide that having your child be poorly focused or overactive is better than having these side effects. Even better, there are alternative therapies which use *no* stimulant drugs.

## OLDER ADULTS AND PRESCRIPTION DRUGS

ADHD is not the only area where prescription drug use is rising. According to data published by the Department of Health and Human Services (HHS), five out of six persons 65 and older are taking at least one medication and almost half of the elderly population takes three or more. Americans over 65 are taking 34 percent of all prescription drugs, and our senior citizens are among the individuals most vulnerable to drug-related complications.

Poisoning is the fastest growing cause of accidental death among seniors, particularly from overdoses of over-the-counter and prescription medication. Drugs in the benzodiazepine family, used to slow brain activity and treat anxiety and sleeplessness, can easily veer off into the danger zone of abuse. These drugs include:

- Diazepam (Valium)
- Chlordiazepoxide hydrochloride (Librium)
- Alprazolam (Xanax)
- Triazolam (Halcion)
- Estazolam (ProSom)

*SIDE EFFECTS FOR THIS CLASS OF DRUGS INCLUDE:*

- Memory loss or forgetfulness
- Excessive sleepiness
- Zombie-like affect
- Frequent falls or stumbling

ANTI-DEPRESSANT DRUGS FOR DEPRESSION

Depression is the one of the more common ailments for which people seek treatment in our office. It affects people of every age from children through the elderly. Unfortunately, we are seldom the initial choice of treatment for this problem. People typically seek relief first with medication from an allopathic doctor with decidedly mixed results.

According to the Georgetown University Medical Center and a Canadian research institute, antidepressant medication may affect the user's immune system in ways that are not yet understood. The U.S. Food and Drug Administration has issued its strongest warning—the black box warning—on the use of *all* antidepressants because of a higher risk of suicide.[171]

Although these medications may have extremely negative side effects, the number of adults and children using the drugs increased by *73 percent* and *50 percent*, respectively, in the decade between 1996 and 2006.

The introduction of a Prozac advertisement in 1998 changed antidepressant marketing. New television and print ads depicting smiling happy faces and showing the general public how a little pill could change their lives. The viewer's impression is that Prozac and other such drugs can increase energy, confidence and assertiveness. However, the ads typically minimize the debilitating side effects including blunting of creativity, lack of sexual drive, reduced appetite, unexpected bursts of anger and aggression or increased tendency to violent suicidal thoughts.[172]

---

[171] Morgan, D. (2009) U.S. family doctors prescribe most mental health drugs. Reuters. Retrieved from:
http://www.reuters.com/article/healthNews/idUSTRE58T0NE200
90930?pageNumber=2&virtualBrandChannel=11604&sp=true
[172] Ahern, G. (2006) Commonly Used Antidepressants May Also Affect Human Immune System. Retrieved
from:http://explore.georgetown.edu/news/?ID=12369&PageTemplate
ID=295

Marketing is a continual positioning effort to penetrate new audiences and sub-segments of the population. All of the major consumer industries are continually looking for new applications and audiences. Pharmaceuticals frequently have a primary and secondary effect. Therefore pharmaceutical companies are famous for adapting drugs from one market to another. Eli Lilly's marketing of Prozac has been expanded in its application from an antidepressant to use in fighting pre-menstrual syndrome, or PMS. Lilly also knows that taking prescriptions daily is a problem for many people and so introduced "Prozac Weekly" to provide a large once-weekly dose to meet those needs.

## SEROTONIN

The neurotransmitter serotonin is found primarily in the gastrointestinal (GI) tract and the central nervous system (CNS). Although approximately *80 percent* of the human body's total serotonin is located in the gut,[173] where it is used to regulate intestinal movements, it is also synthesized in serotonergic neurons in the CNS where it controls the regulation of mood, appetite, sleep, muscle contraction, and some cognitive functions including memory and learning.

We know that part of the mechanism that regulates serotonin levels is the reabsorption of a portion of it into the cell from which it's released into the synapse.

---

[173] King, M.W.(2009) Serotonin. *The Medical Biochemistry Page.* Indiana University School of Medicine.

This mechanism is called Serotonin reuptake.[174] The class of drugs that modify this mechanism in an attempt to increase overall serotonin levels is *Selective Serotonin Reuptake Inhibitors*, or SSRIs.

According to a study published in September 2009 in the Archives of General Psychiatry, at least 27 million Americans take antidepressants; more than double the number who took them in the mid-1990s. Paxil and Prozac, the most commonly prescribed antidepressants, are SSRIs.[175]

Not only do these SSRIs flood the body with serotonin, they also interfere with the body's ability to metabolize serotonin, resulting in a buildup of toxic amounts after prolonged use.
In other words, an SSRI antidepressant impairs the ability of cells to metabolize serotonin, not only in the brain, but, since serotonin is widely distributed throughout the body, in the rest of the body as well.

For years, research that showed SSRI antidepressants to be dangerous and nearly useless was kept hidden, while the studies published and presented to potential prescribers painted a glowing picture of success. The tactics worked well. We would be hard-pressed today to find someone who does not have a family member or friend labeled mentally ill and taking drugs like Prozac,

---

[174] Berger M, Gray JA, Roth BL (2009) The expanded biology of serotonin. *Annu. Rev. Med.* 60: 355–66. doi:10.1146/annurev.med.60.042307.110802
[175] Angst. J., Azorin, J.M., Bowden, C.L., Perugi, G., Vieta, E., Gamma, A., et al. (2011) Prevalence and Characteristics of Undiagnosed Bipolar Disorders in Patients With a Major Depressive Episode: The BRIDGE Study. *Archives of general psychiatry*, 68(8), 791-798. PMID: 21810644

Paxil, Zoloft, Lexapro and Celexa, or their chemical cousins Effexor, Cymbalta and Wellbutrin.[176]

The Senate Finance Committee under its then-ranking Republican, Senator Charles Grassley, investigated GlaxoSmithKline, because of new revelations in a report filed in litigation showing that the company manipulated the numbers on adverse events related to suicide in clinical trials back in 1989. The manipulated data made it appear that Paxil did not increase the risk of patients experiencing suicidal behavior when, in fact, trial subjects on Paxil were *eight times* more likely to attempt or commit suicide than patients taking placebos.[177]

On February 6, 2007, Dr. David Healy, an Irish psychiatrist and professor in Psychological Medicine at Cardiff University School of Medicine, Wales, published a commentary entitled, *Why you should never trust new wonder drugs*. Dr. Healy commented that through lawsuits, research has finally been revealed to the public that showed that the pharmaceutical companies knew that these drugs were statistically responsible for an increased risk of suicide and that they were only slightly more effective than a placebo. Moreover, "...[t]he scientific literature, the very place doctors would look for a warning," he writes, "contained barely a hint of problems."

---

[176] Healy, D. (2003) *Let Them Eat Prozac*. Ontario, Canada: The Canadian Association of University Teachers
[177] Grassley, Sen. Charles (2008) Grassley seeks FDA scrutiny of Paxil and suicide risk. United States Senate Committee on Finance. Retrieved from:
http://finance.senate.gov/press/Gpress/2008/prg061208.pdf

Healy's website
(http://www.healyprozac.com/context.htm) contains
court papers and other documents that support the
allegations he has made about SSRI research.

*SEROTONIN SYNDROME*

Another effect of taking SSRIs is so-called "serotonin
syndrome," a potentially life-threatening reaction
caused by excessive levels of serotonin. This problem is
multiplied when taking more than just the triggering
SSRI medication. For example, migraine medicines
called triptans together with antidepressants can
produce the syndrome. [178] Other potential triggers
include older antidepressants called monoamine
oxidase inhibitors (MAOIs). Meperidine (Demerol, a
painkiller), dextromethorphan (found in over-the-
counter cough medicines) and illegal drugs such as
Ecstasy and LSD have also been associated with
Serotonin syndrome. Symptoms occur within minutes
to hours, and may include:

- Agitation or restlessness
- Diarrhea
- Fast heartbeat
- Hallucinations
- Raised body temperature
- Loss of coordination
- Nausea

---

[178] US Food and Drug Administration. FDA Public Health Advisory:
Combined Use of 5-Hydroxytryptamine Receptor Agonists (Triptans),
Selective Serotonin Reuptake Inhibitors (SSRIs) or Selective
Serotonin/Norepinephrine Reuptake Inhibitors (SNRIs) May Result in
Life-threatening Serotonin Syndrome. Rockville, MD: Center for Drug
Evaluation and Research; July 19, 2006.

- Overactive reflexes
- Rapid changes in blood pressure
- Vomiting

## SSRI DISCONTINUATION SYNDROME

Serotonin Syndrome isn't the only potential issue. The serotonin supply that is being depleted from the cells as the SSRI inhibits its absorption can also cause a problem.

*SSRI Discontinuation Syndrome* results as the dose of the drug is reduced or discontinued.

SSRI's are split into two categories: long-acting and short-acting. For example, Prozac is a longer-acting SSRI. Paxil, Effexor, Zoloft and Luvox are short-acting. The short-acting SSRIs, when discontinued or when the dosage is reduced, produce an "anticholinergic rebound," which is an production interruption of the key neurotransmitter *acetylcholine*. (Remember, acetylcholine is the neurotransmitter that sees significant use when a person is under greater stress). [179]

Symptoms include:

- Headache
- Diarrhea
- Nausea
- Vomiting
- Chills
- Dizziness

---

[179] Tamam L, Ozpoyraz N (2002). "Selective serotonin reuptake inhibitor discontinuation syndrome: a review". *Adv Ther* **19** (1): 17–26. doi:10.1007/BF02850015

- Fatigue
- Insomnia
- Agitation
- Impaired concentration
- Vivid dreams
- De-personalization (feeling disconnected from oneself)
- Irritability
- Suicidal thoughts

These symptoms are from the body struggling to adapt to the absence of a chemical which had been present in unusually high amounts. Such symptoms usually last from one to seven weeks and then decline.

Double-blind controlled studies now indicate that 35-78% of patients who stop abruptly after five weeks or more of treatment with SSRIs or titrate down in increments of at least 10mg, will develop one or more of the discontinuation symptoms.[180]

When allowed to run its course, SSRI discontinuation syndrome duration is variable (one to several weeks) and ranges in intensity from mild-to-moderate in most patients to extremely distressing in a small number.

Other types of antidepressants include selective norepinephrine inhibitors (SNRIs) which are similar to SSRIs and include venlafaxine (Effexor) and duloxetine (Cymbalta). Another antidepressant in common use is bupropion (Wellbutrin). Bupropion works on the

---

[180] Michelson D, Fava M, Amsterdam J et al. (April 2000). "Interruption of selective serotonin reuptake inhibitor treatment. Double-blind, placebo-controlled trial". Br J Psychiatry 176 (4): 363–8. doi:10.1192/bjp.176.4.363. PMID 10827885.

neurotransmitter dopamine and is unique in that it does not fit into any specific drug type.

## BIPOLAR DISORDER

Bipolar disorder is a psychiatric illness that typically involves manic mood swings from incredible highs to devastating lows. Until very recently this disorder was only observed in adults. The relatively new practice of diagnosing young children with this disorder could have disastrous results, as the use of psychotropic drugs to treat bipolar disorder is common.

## NON-DRUG ALTERNATIVES

The promise of a wonder drug that cures all ills is obviously appealing. After all, addressing the root cause of an issue can take time and work. But for those that are looking for a permanent change, drugs are not the answer. And as we have seen in this chapter, they can cause more problems than they cure.

Although I am one of the owners of a company that uses non-drug approaches for both ADHD and depression/anxiety, I can say that my opinion on this matter is not based on financials. It is based instead on our results with the people who walk through our door every day.

Many of our patients come to us after struggling with the decision to use medication. Others have tried medications that did not cure the underlying cause of the problem, and are now struggling with the *medications'* effects, or they find they are unable to discontinue the medication without significant withdrawal symptoms.

Still, not every patient is a candidate for non-drug therapy.

It requires that the patient have a desire to heal and a willingness to complete the therapy regimen. Those patients who qualify for our therapies experience relief of their symptoms, control over their own bodies and a whole new outlook on life.

## PERFORMANCE-ENHANCING DRUGS

Competition can create a fierce drive to win. This can result in both beneficial and detrimental effects on the competitor. Winning can bring power and glory, and it is because of this that some will always look for a magic potion to bolster their performance.

Unfortunately, these substances also compromise the ethical standards inherent in sport, not to mention the competitor's health. Although performance-enhancing drugs in professional sports are banned, many people are concerned that their use continues. Even worse, young athletes will emulate winning sports figures, even to their use of performance-enhancing drugs.

Why would anyone risk using these drugs? It's easy: in our society, star athletes are celebrities. They can earn enormous amounts of money and enjoy fame, if not notoriety. However, most of these athletes know they have relatively short careers in which they are at their best.

Athletes know that training is the best and safest path to victory. But they can't avoid the constant messages from our drug-dominated society that drugs are an effective shortcut to higher performance, even at the cost of their health and athletic careers.

Even as far back as ancient Greece, athletes were often willing to take any preparation that would offer improved performance. However, it appears that drug use has increased since the 1960s. For example, one notorious example is the Canadian sprinter Ben Johnson. After setting world records prior to the 1988 Seoul Olympics, he tested positive for anabolic steroids and was stripped of his gold medal. Thereafter, he was caught *twice more* with banned substances in his tested blood.

Motives for using drugs in sports—"doping"—include the physical (e.g. better performance, pain control), psychological (e.g. anxiety, pressure, stress, fatigue) and social (e.g. pressure on result, group acceptance). These motives are primarily based upon human and social behaviors, emotions and personality.

The limbic system of the brain controls instinctive behavior, emotions and motivation. Neurotransmitters like adrenaline, noradrenaline, dopamine, serotonin and GABA are involved in the control of many emotional and mental states. Most of the psychoactive drugs work by changing either the *metabolism* of the neurotransmitters, or the specific *receptor* sensitivity for these neurotransmitters.

A special group of neurotransmitters, endorphins, are structurally similar to opioids, are involved in sensations of pain and pleasure. Dopamine and serotonin influence the "reward system" in the brain. All drugs that artificially create a dependency increase the amount of dopamine in the reward system and help increase pleasure, reduce pain and/or reduce stress. [181]

Extended drug use may cause tolerance, dependence, addiction or withdrawal effects. *Tolerance* is a compensating mechanism that results in a gradual reduction in the effect of drugs. *Drug dependence* occurs when continued consumption of a drug is needed to prevent or diminish the physical or psychological disturbances of withdrawal (abstinence syndrome). [182] *Physical dependence* occurs when the body is deprived of a drug. Deprivation leads to physical symptoms such as pain, severe tremors or convulsions.

Continued stimulation of the reward system can create the development of *psychological dependence*. Psychological dependence can last much longer and be much stronger than physical dependence. This is one reason that addiction can cause such a compulsive need for drugs despite the adverse consequences.[183]

Athletes are at risk for all of these effects when taking drugs to enhance performance. An athlete may want to:

- Build mass and strength of muscles and/or bones

---

[181] Sapolsky, R. (2005) *Biology and Human Behavior: The Neurological Origins of Individuality, 2nd edition.* Chantilly, VA: The Teaching Company.

[182] Lehmann, P. (2002). *Coming off Psychiatric Drugs*. Germany: Peter Lehmann Publishing. ISBN 1-891408-98-4.

[183] Rothman, et al. (2001)Amphetamine-Type Central Nervous System Stimulants Release Norepinepehrine more Potently than they Release Dopamine and Serotonin. *Synapse 39*, 32-41

- Increase delivery of oxygen to exercising tissues
- Suppress or mask pain
- Stimulate the body
- Relax
- Reduce weight
- Hide the use of other drugs

The following is a list of some of the more popular performance-enhancing drugs being used by athletes to build mass and strength:

- Anabolic-androgenic steroids
- Beta-2 agonists
- Human chorionic gonadotropin (hCG)
- Luteinizing hormone (LH)
- Human growth hormone (hGH)
- Insulin-like growth factor (IGF-1)
- Insulin

## ANABOLIC-ANDROGENIC STEROIDS

A steroid is a chemical substance derived from cholesterol. There are several principal steroid hormones: testosterone in the male and estrogen and progesterone in the female. *Catabolic steroids* break down tissue, and *anabolic steroids* build up tissue. Anabolic steroids build muscle and bone mass primarily by stimulating the muscle and bone cells to make new protein.[184]

---

[184] Powers, M. (2005) Performance-Enhancing Drugs in Houglum,J., Harrelson,G.L. &Leaver-Dunn, D., *Principles of Pharmacology for Athletic Trainers*, SLACK Incorporated. ISBN 1-55642-594-5, p. 330

After a steroid is ingested, it is distributed to many regions of the brain, including the hypothalamus. The hypothalamus produces testosterone, which controls appetite, blood pressure, mood and reproductive ability. Steroids change the level of testosterone in the body, and because testosterone plays a role in many body functions, this can result in many effects seen with steroid abuse.

Testosterone has two main effects on the body:

- Anabolic effects promote muscle building.
- Androgenic effects are responsible for male traits, such as facial hair and a deeper voice.

Steroids can also disrupt the functioning of neurons in the limbic system, that part of the brain responsible for emotional regulation. This disruption can lead to aggressive behavior, mood swings, violent behavior, impairment of judgment, and even psychotic symptoms like personality changes or paranoia.

Some athletes take straight testosterone to boost their performance. Frequently, the anabolic-androgenic steroids used by athletes are synthetic modifications of testosterone. These hormones have approved medical uses, although improving athletic performance is not one of them. They can be taken as pills, injections or topical treatments.[185] Common anabolic-androgenic steroids include:

---

[185] Hoberman JM, Yesalis CE (1995) The history of synthetic testosterone. *Scientific American* **272** (2): 76–81. doi:10.1038/scientificamerican0295-76. PMID 7817189

- Testosterone
- Dihydrotestosterone
- Androstenedione ("Andro")
- Dehydroepiandrosterone (DHEA)
- Clostebol
- Nandrolone

Why are these drugs so appealing to athletes? Besides making muscles bigger, anabolic-androgenic steroids may help athletes recover from a hard workout more quickly by reducing the amount of muscle damage that occurs during training or competition. In addition, some athletes like the aggressive feelings they get when they take the drugs.

## DESIGNER STEROIDS

A particularly dangerous class of anabolic androgenic steroids has emerged since 2002. These so-called "designer" drugs are synthetic steroids that have been illicitly created to be undetectable in current drug tests. They are made specifically for athletes and have no approved medical use. Because of this, they haven't been tested or approved by the Food and Drug Administration (FDA) and represent a particular health threat to athletes.[186]

---

[186] King, L.A. (2009) New drugs coming our way - what are they and how do we detect them? EMCDDA Conference, Lisbon, 6–8 May 2009 http://www.emcdda.europa.eu/attachements.cfm/att_78745_EN_4 _King.pps

Designer steroids include:

- Tetrahydrogestrinone (THG)
- Desoxymethyltestosterone (Madol)
- Norbolethone (Genabol)

## *RISKS*

Many athletes take anabolic-androgenic steroids at doses that are much higher than those prescribed for medical reasons, and most of what is known about the drugs' effects on athletes comes from observing these users. It is impossible for researchers to design studies that would accurately test the effects of large doses of steroids on athletes, because giving test participants such high doses would be unethical. Thus, the effects of taking anabolic-androgenic steroids at very high doses haven't been well studied.

Anabolic-androgenic steroids come with serious physical side effects as well.

Men may develop:

- Prominent breasts
- Baldness
- Shrunken testicles
- Infertility

Women may develop:

- A deeper voice
- An enlarged clitoris
- Increased body hair
- Baldness

Both men and women might experience:

- Severe acne
- Liver abnormalities and tumors
- Increased low-density lipoprotein (LDL) cholesterol (the "bad" cholesterol)
- Decreased high-density lipoprotein (HDL) cholesterol (the "good" cholesterol)
- Aggressive behaviors, rage or violence
- Psychiatric disorders, such as depression
- Drug dependence
- Infections or diseases such as HIV or hepatitis if you're injecting the drugs
- Inhibited growth and development, and risk of future health problems if you're a teenager

In the past 20 years, more effective law enforcement in the United States has pushed much of the illegal steroid industry into the black market. This poses additional health risks because the drugs are either manufactured in other countries and smuggled in or manufactured in clandestine US labs. In either case, they aren't subject to government safety standards and could be impure or mislabeled.

## BETA-2 AGONISTS

Beta-2-adrenoreceptor (beta-2) agonists act as bronchodilators. The drugs stimulate the airways in the lungs (bronchi) to open wider, permitting more air to pass.[187]

The drugs are used primarily by asthmatics who suffer from insufficient air supply to the lungs because of narrowing of the bronchi. Athletes use beta-2 agonists to increase the infusion of air in their lungs thus improving their athletic performance.

Beta-2 agonists include:

- Salbutamol
- Salmeterol
- Terbutaline
- Eformoterol

These drugs mimic the effects of adrenaline and noradrenaline that are naturally produced in the body. Bronchial dilation is an intended effect from these natural substances to prepare the body to react for action (the "fight or flight" reaction).[188]

The beta-2 agonists interact with a particular receptor on the surface of the lung tissue as they enter the lung bronchi. It is this interaction with beta-2 receptors that stimulates the expansion of the bronchi.

These drugs are typically delivered to the lungs using an inhaler, although they can be delivered by injection,

---

[187] National Asthma Education and Prevention Program. Bethesda, MD: NIH; Expert Panel Report 2: Guidelines for the diagnosis and management of asthma; pp. 245–253. Publication number 97–4051.
[188] Giembycz, M.A.(2000) *Phosphodiesterase 4 inhibitors and the treatment of asthma: where are we now and where do we go from here? Drugs 2000;59:193–212*

as a vapor produced by a nebulizer, as a tablet, or in syrup form.

Beta-2 agonists have become a concern in sports. At high doses, the drug can act as an anabolic agent to promote gain in weight, mainly in the form of muscle. However, in 2006, the World Anti-Doping Agency ruled that select beta-2 agonists (salbutamol, salmeterol, terbutaline, and eformoterol) in inhalation form were allowed for use in those athletes who were asthmatic only to prevent or treat exercise-induced asthma or bronchial constriction. Oral and injected forms of beta-2 agonists are still illegal. If levels of beta-2 agonist are detected, an athlete must demonstrate that the drug was used for asthma.[189]

## EFFECTS ON PERFORMANCE

Inhaled forms of Beta-2 agonists used for the treatment of asthma have no performance-enhancing effect. However, when administered by injection or tablet form they are thought to have anabolic effects (increased muscle mass, reduced body fat percentage and faster recovery rates). [190]

---

[189] The world anti-doping code. The 2009 prohibited list. Montreal, Canada: International Standard; 2009.
[190] Nijkamp, F.P., Engels, F., Henricks, P.A., Van Oosterhout, A.J.(1997) f β-adrenergic receptor regulation in lungs and its implications for physiological responses. *Physiol Rev 1992;72:323–367.*

## SIDE-EFFECTS OF BETA-2-AGONISTS [191]

- Tachycardia (rapid heartbeat)
- Palpitations (abnormal/irregular heartbeat)
- Headaches
- Tremors
- Nervousness
- Sweating
- Nausea
- Vomiting

## HUMAN CHORIONIC GONADOTROPIN (HCG)

HCG is a glycoprotein hormone produced during pregnancy by the embryo shortly after conception and later in larger amounts by the placenta. The function of HCG during pregnancy is to maintain the corpus luteum (an endocrine structure found in the ovaries, vital for the maintenance of a pregnancy) and causing it to secrete progesterone (this causes the uterus to develop a thick layer of capillaries to help sustain the fetus).

When used with anabolic androgenic steroids, hCG can help the male athlete maintain and restore testicular

---

[191] National Institutes of Health (2007). National Asthma Education and Prevention Program Expert Panel Report 3: Guidelines for the Diagnosis and Management of Asthma (NIH Publication No. 08–5846). Retrieved from:
http://www.nhlbi.nih.gov/guidelines/asthma/asthgdln.htm.

size as well as normal testosterone production affected by the steroids.[192]

Because it is produced naturally in women, restrictions don't apply to women athletes. However, due to its use with various anabolic-androgenic steroids, its use by male athletes is illegal.[193]

## SIDE-EFFECTS OF HUMAN CHORIONIC GONADOTROPHIN

Side-effects from hCG can be seen when it is used for too long and/or too high a dose. The resulting rise in natural testosterone will eventually inhibit its own production in the hypothalamus and pituitary gland.

The principal side-effect of HCG is gynecomastia (the development of abnormally large mammary glands in males due to increased levels of estrogen.

The combination of HCG and Anabolic Steroids can cause:[194]

- Headaches
- Depression
- Edema (swelling caused by fluid within the body's tissues)

---

[192] Williams, L. (May 8, 2009). *San Francisco Chronicle*. Retrieved from http://articles.sfgate.com/2009-05-08/sports/17199689_1_hcg-steroid-users-steroid-cycle

[193] Cole LA (2009)New discoveries on the biology and detection of human chorionic gonadotropin. *Reprod. Biol. Endocrinol.* **7**: 8. doi:10.1186/1477-7827-7-8. PMID 19171054

[194] van Breda, E., Keizer, H.A., Kuipers, H. & Wolffenbuttel, B.H. (April 2003) Androgenic anabolic steroid use and severe hypothalamic-pituitary dysfunction: a case study. *Int J Sports Med* 24 (3): 195–6. doi:10.1055/s-2003-39089

## LUTEINIZING HORMONE (LH)

LH is a hormone produced by the anterior lobe of the pituitary gland that stimulates ovulation and the development of the corpus luteum in the female and the production of testosterone by the interstitial cells of the testes in the male.

Its use is considered equivalent to testosterone and is therefore on the World Anti-Doping Agency's 2005 Prohibited List. Although no general side effects exist, any possible side effects might be similar to those of anabolic steroids.[195]

## HUMAN GROWTH HORMONE

Human Growth Hormone (hGH) is a naturally occurring protein hormone produced by the pituitary gland and is important for normal human growth and development, especially in children and teenagers.

Low hGH levels in children and teenagers result in dwarfism. Excessive hGH levels increase muscle mass by stimulating protein synthesis, strengthen bones by stimulating bone growth and reduce body fat by stimulating the breakdown of fat cells. Use of hGH has become increasingly popular because it is difficult to detect.

---

[195] Louvet J, Harman S, Ross G (1975) Effects of human chorionic gonadotropin, human interstitial cell stimulating hormone and human follicle-stimulating hormone on ovarian weights in estrogen-primed hypophysectomized immature female rats. *Endocrinology* **96** (5): 1179–86. doi:10.1210/endo-96-5-1179

Side effects include:[196]

- Overgrowth of hands, feet, and face (acromegaly) because of the increased muscle and bone development in these parts
- Enlarged internal organs, especially heart, kidneys, tongue and liver
- Heart problems

## INSULIN-LIKE GROWTH FACTOR

Insulin-like Growth Factor (IGF-1), is also known as somatomedin-C. It is a naturally occurring protein that helps in the action of hGH. It also stimulates protein synthesis and reduces fat. Excessive IGF-1 increases muscle and bone mass.

Side effects include:[197]

- Low blood sugar (hypoglycemia)
- Effects similar to hGH.

## INSULIN

Insulin is a natural protein hormone produced by the pancreas. It is important in the metabolism of sugars, starches, fats, and proteins. In athletes, insulin

---

[196] Powers M (2005) Performance-Enhancing Drugs. in Leaver-Dunn, D.; Houglum, J.; et al *Principles of Pharmacology for Athletic Trainers*. Slack Incorporated. pp. 331–332.

[197] Gunnell, D., Miller, L.L., Rogers, I. & Holly, J.M. (2005) Association of insulin-like growth factor I and insulin-like growth factor-binding protein-3 with intelligence quotient among 8- to 9-year-old children in the Avon Longitudinal Study of Parents and Children. *Pediatrics*. Nov;116(5):e681-6. PMID 16263982

combined with anabolic steroids or hGH increases muscle mass by stimulating protein synthesis. Side effects are mainly low blood sugar associated with shaking, nausea and weakness, but excessive hypoglycemia can lead to coma and death. [198]

## INCREASING OXYGEN IN TISSUES

In addition to taking drugs that build mass and strength, some athletes take drugs and engage in practices that increase the amount of oxygen in tissues, including protein hormones, artificial oxygen carriers and blood doping.

### PROTEIN HORMONES

Erythropoietin (EPO) is a hormone normally produced by the kidneys, which regulates red blood cell production in the bone marrow. It is naturally occurring and is secreted by the kidneys during low-oxygen conditions. EPO stimulates the bone marrow stem cells to make red blood cells, which increase the delivery of oxygen to the kidneys.

Endurance athletes, such as those who compete in marathons, cycling or cross-country skiing, can use EPO to increase their oxygen supply by as much as seven to 10 percent. EPO is difficult to detect. The increased red cell density caused by EPO, however, can thicken the blood. The thickened blood does not flow well through the blood vessels. To pump the thickened

---

[198] Sonksen, P.H. & Sonksen, J. (2000) Insulin: understanding its action in health and disease. *British Journal of Anesthesia* **85** 69–79.

blood, the heart must work harder, which increases the chances of heart attack and stroke. [199]

## ARTIFICIAL OXYGEN CARRIERS

Artificial Oxygen Carriers are man-made substances that can do the work of hemoglobin, the oxygen-carrying protein in the blood. They are normally used for treating breathing difficulties in premature infants, patients with severe lung injuries and in deep-sea divers.

Blood is composed of plasma, platelets, white blood cells, and red blood cells. Of these, red blood cells (erythrocytes) are the most relevant to blood oxygenation enhancement. Erythrocytes travel through the body delivering oxygen and removing carbon dioxide. Their red color is due to a chemical protein called hemoglobin, the substance that allows them to transport gases.

As blood passes through the lungs, oxygen molecules attach to the hemoglobin, and as blood passes through the body's tissues, the hemoglobin releases that oxygen to the cells. [200] It is this oxygen that prevents the conversion of pyruvic acid to lactic acid, thereby delaying the onset of muscle fatigue and prolonging an athlete's ability to perform.[201]

[199] Höke, A. (2005). *Erythropoietin and the Nervous System*. Berlin: Springer.
[200] The Franklin Institute Online. The Heart: An Online Exploration. http://sln.fi.edu/
[201] Rogol, A.D. (1993) Hormonal ergogenic aids. *J. of Sport Rehab.*, Champaign (Ill.), 2 (1993), 2, pp. 128-140

Artificially enhancing blood oxygenation increases an individual's hemoglobin concentration above normally occurring levels. This can be done in two ways:

- Blood transfusions to stimulate increased hemoglobin levels in the blood
- Using chemicals to increase the blood's ability to carry extra oxygen.

Artificial Oxygen Carriers include:

- Perfluorocarbons, synthetic- or modified-hemoglobin
- Liposome-encased hemoglobin (artificial red cells).

## BLOOD DOPING

Blood doping is the practice of infusing whole blood into an athlete in order to increase oxygen delivery to the tissues. This is a relatively simple means of enhancing an athlete's endurance by increasing the amount of oxygen-carrying red cells in the blood stream.

This method is undetectable, but it has one downside: the anemia that results when the blood is extracted makes it hard for the athlete to train. For this reason athletes often chose to use donor blood from the same blood type. Unlike using your own blood, using donor blood is detectable.

Blood doping is believed to have entered sport in the 1970s but was not made illegal until 1986. Before then it was in vogue among middle- and long-distance runners. It is still in use today as Floyd Landis, Tour de

France winner, confessed to blood doping and accused famed cyclist Lance Armstrong of blood doping as well.[202] As of this writing, Armstrong has abandoned his contest of the charges against him; he has been stripped of his seven Tour de France wins and banned from cycling.

## SIDE EFFECTS

No matter the perceived benefits, blood doping isn't just against the rules, it's dangerous. Transfusions done at home, for example, can incur the risks of contracting blood-borne diseases and becoming ill from bacteria growing in poorly stored blood.[203]

Doping can also make the blood dangerously thick. When hemoglobin is too high, you can run into many complications, the worst of which is clotting.

An athlete who infuses his own blood may cause infection or cardiovascular problems because of the increased blood volume (high blood pressure, blood clots, heart failure and stroke). An athlete who uses someone else's blood also runs the risk of acquiring viral infections such as HIV/AIDS. [204]

---

[202] Urhausen, A., Albers T. & Kindermann, W. (2003) Reversibility of the effects on blood cells, lipids, liver function and hormones in former anabolic–androgenic steroid abusers. *The Journal of Steroid Biochemistry and Molecular Biology*. Volume 84, Issues 2-3, February 2003, Pages 369-375

[203] Blajchman M. (2002) Incidence and significance of the bacterial contamination of blood components. *Dev Biol* (Basel) 108: 59-67.

[204] Fotheringham, W. (22 September 2004). It can kill, but blood doping is in vogue again. *The Guardian*. London. http://www.guardian.co.uk/sport/2004/sep/22/cycling.cycling.

# Drugs for Pain

Athletes are more susceptible to injuries and pain when training and performing in competitive and professional world-class sports. Sometimes, athletes try to mask their injury pain with drugs, including narcotics, protein hormones, cortisone and local anesthetics.

## Narcotics

Narcotics are used to treat pain and include substances such as morphine, methadone and heroin. They are highly addictive and the "high" associated with their use can also impair mental abilities (judgment, balance and concentration).

Potential benefits to athletes from the use of narcotics include euphoria and a heightened pain threshold. The downside of narcotic use includes false feeling of invincibility, illusions of athletic prowess beyond an athlete's inherent ability, failure to recognize injury, and physical and psychological dependence.

All narcotic analgesics including codeine and dihydrocodeine heroin (diacetylmorphine) are banned by the International Olympic committee (IOC) as well as the US Olympic Committee (USOC).

## Protein Hormones

Adrenocorticotrophic hormone (ACTH) is a naturally occurring hormone that is secreted by the pituitary gland and stimulates the production of hormones from the adrenal cortex. These adrenal cortex hormones are important in reducing inflammation in injuries and allergic responses. Athletes use this hormone to mask injuries.

## Side effects

Side effects for use of these hormones include:

- Stomach irritation
- Ulcers
- Mental irritation
- Long-term weakening of bones and muscles

### CORTISONE

Cortisone is one of the adrenal cortex hormones. Clinically, it is injected to reduce inflammation in injuries and allergic responses. The advantages and side effects of its use are the same as with Adrenocorticotrophic hormone (ACTH).

### LOCAL ANESTHETICS

Local anesthetics, similar to those used by your dentist or doctor, are used to mask pain in the short-term without impairing mental abilities. They include:

- Novocaine
- Procaine
- Lidocaine
- Lignocaine

Athletes may use them so that they can compete while injured. The major problem with their use is the possibility of further damage to the injured area.

# DRUGS FOR STIMULATION, RELAXATION AND WEIGHT CONTROL

Many athletes live within strict social and dietary guidelines. To cope with stress, general fatigue and weight, many athletes turn to stimulating, relaxing and weight controlling drugs.

## *STIMULANTS*

Stimulants are generally used to help athletes stay alert, reduce fatigue and maintain aggressiveness. They act on the body to make the heart beat faster, the lungs breathe faster and the brain work faster (if not better). Stimulants include caffeine, amphetamines and cocaine.

Stimulants act by altering levels of the neurotransmitters dopamine and norepinephrine in the synapses in various brain regions. Because methamphetamine has a similar chemical structure to dopamine and norepinephrine, it can be picked up by neurons that normally recycle these neurotransmitters. It can also enter neurons by passing directly across the cell membrane. Once these stimulants enter a neuron, the neuron releases large amounts of both dopamine and norepinephrine into the synapse. The high concentrations of dopamine result in feelings of euphoria and pleasure.

Norepinephrine most likely causes the alertness seen with stimulant use; however when a person stops using stimulants, the reduction of dopamine in the synapse results in intense cravings for the drug.

## Side Effects

- Nervousness
- Shaking
- Irregular heartbeat
- High blood pressure
- Convulsions and
- Sudden death.

## *RELAXANTS*

Relaxants come in various forms, including alcohol, prescription drugs such as beta-blockers, and cannabinoids, such as marijuana.

Alcohol is commonly used for relaxation because it reduces activity in the brain and nervous system. While it may help an athlete relax and cope with the pressures of competition, it can also significantly impair mental functions, such as judgment, balance, and coordination. It is restricted in the Olympics and banned altogether in certain events.

Beta-blockers are commonly prescribed to treat high blood pressure by causing the heart to slow down and blood vessels to relax and dilate. Athletes who require steady hands in competition, such as those competing in archery or shooting events, may use them. Possible side effects include lower than normal blood pressure (hypotension), slow heart rate and fatigue.

Cannabinoids, primarily marijuana and hashish, have no clinical value, but have recently seen increased use for pain relief in terminally ill cancer patients. Cannabinoids cause hallucinations, induce drowsiness, increase the heart rate and impair mental functions, such as judgment, balance, coordination and memory.

## WEIGHT CONTROL

### DIURETICS

Diuretics are commonly prescribed to treat high blood pressure and are often found in diet pills. Diuretics act on the kidney to increase the flow of urine. Diuretics are also used to mask the use of other drugs. Because they increase the amount of urine output, they dilute the concentration of other drugs in the urine.[205]

Diuretics change the body's natural balance of electrolytes—fluids and salts—and can lead to dehydration. This loss of water can decrease an athlete's weight, helping him or her to compete in a lighter weight class, preferred by many athletes. Diuretics may also help athletes pass drug tests by diluting their urine.

Diuretics are used by athletes whose events have weight restrictions, such as weightlifting, boxing, wrestling, rowing and horse racing (the jockey's weight is the critical value, not that of the horse).[206]

---

[205] Mutschler, E. (1995) Drug actions: basic principles and therapeutic aspects. Stuttgart, German: *Medpharm Scientific Pub.* p. 460.
[206] British Journal of Pharmacology (2010)The abuse of diuretics as performance-enhancing drugs and masking agents in sport doping: pharmacology, toxicology and analysis, 2010-09.

Some of the most common diuretics include:

- Acetazolamide (Diamox)
- Spironolactone (Aldactone)
- Furosemide (Lasix)

If diuretics are taken at a dose above the medically recommended dose, the adverse effects may be significant. These include:

- Dehydration
- Muscle cramps
- Exhaustion
- Dizziness
- Potassium deficiency
- Heart arrhythmias
- Drop in blood pressure
- Death

## NUTRITIONAL SUPPLEMENTS

Illegal drugs aren't the only way athletes are enhancing their performance. So-called "natural supplements" are also being used instead of, or in addition to, performance-enhancing drugs. Supplements are available over-the-counter as liquids, powders or pills.

Supplements are considered food and not drugs by the FDA. This means supplement manufacturers are not required to conform to the same production safety standards as drug manufacturers and not all supplements are created equal. It is common to find supplements that have been diluted or contaminated with other substances, which may inadvertently lead to a positive test for performance-enhancing drugs. [207]

## CREATINE

The most popular supplement among athletes is creatine monohydrate. Creatine is a naturally occurring compound produced by your body that helps your muscles release energy. [208]

Scientific research indicates that creatine may have some athletic benefit by producing small gains in short-term bursts of power. Its benefits include:

- Helping muscles make and circulate more adenosine triphosphate (ATP), which stores and transports energy in cells, and is used for quick, explosive bursts of activity, such as weightlifting or sprinting
- Delaying muscle fatigue

There's no evidence that creatine enhances performance in aerobic or endurance sports.

Your liver produces about 0.07 ounces (2 grams) of creatine each day. Creatine is also obtained from the meat in your diet. Creatine is stored in your muscles, and the levels are relatively easily maintained. Because your kidneys remove excess creatine, the value of

---

[207] Poortmans JR, F. M. (September 2000) Adverse effects of creatine supplementation: fact or fiction?. *Sports Medicine* **30** (3): 155–70. doi:10.2165/00007256-200030030-00002. PMID 10999421
[208] Allen, P.J. (May 2012) Creatine metabolism and psychiatric disorders: Does creatine supplementation have therapeutic value?. *Neurosci Biobehav Rev* 36 (5): 1442–62. doi:10.1016/j.neubiorev.2012.03.005

supplements to someone who already has adequate muscle creatine content is questionable.[209]

Possible side effects of creatine that can decrease athletic performance include:

- Stomach cramps
- Muscle cramps
- Nausea
- Diarrhea
- Weight gain

Weight gain is sought after by athletes who want to increase body mass, but with prolonged creatine use, weight gain is more likely to be from water retention than an increase in muscle mass. Water is drawn into your muscle tissue, away from other parts of your body. This puts you at risk of dehydration.

High-dose creatine use may potentially damage your kidneys and liver. [210]Although it appears safe for adults to use creatine at the doses recommended by manufacturers, the effects of long-term creatine use are unknown, especially in teens or children. The American College of Sports Medicine advises those under 18 years old not to take creatine. The Mayo Clinic also warns that creatine has been associated with asthmatic symptoms and advises against consumption by all with known allergies. They list the side effects of creatine as:

---

[209] Poortmans JR, F.M. JR (December 2006) Side effects of creatine supplementation in athletes. *International Journal of Sports Physiology and Performance* 1 (4): 311–23. PMID 19124889.
[210] Gross, J.L., de Azevedo, M.J., Silveiro, S.P., Canani, L.H., Caramori, M.L. & Zelmanovitz ,T. (January 2005) Diabetic nephropathy: diagnosis, prevention, and treatment. *Diabetes Care* 28 (1): 164–76. doi:10.2337/diacare.28.1.164

- Gastrointestinal symptoms, including loss of appetite, stomach discomfort, diarrhea, or nausea
- Muscle cramps or muscle breakdown, leading to muscle tears or discomfort
- Strains and sprains have been reported due to enthusiastic increases in workout regimens once starting creatine
- Weight gain and increased body mass may occur
- Heat intolerance
- Fever
- Dehydration
- Reduced blood volume, or electrolyte imbalances (and resulting seizures) may occur

Those with kidney disease should avoid use of this supplement. Also, it is noteworthy that liver function may be altered, and caution is advised in those with underlying liver disease. Caution is also advised for those with diabetes or hypoglycemia.

It has been theorized that creatine may alter the activities of insulin. Caution is also advised in patients with diabetes or hypoglycemia, and in those taking drugs, herbs, or supplements that affect blood sugar. Serum glucose levels may need to be monitored by a healthcare professional, and medication adjustments may be necessary.

Long-term administration of large quantities of creatine has also been reported to increase the production of formaldehyde, which may potentially cause serious unwanted side effects. [211]

Creatine may also increase the risk of compartment syndrome of the lower leg, a condition characterized by pain in the lower leg associated with inflammation and ischemia (diminished blood flow), which may result in a need for emergency surgery.

Reports of other side effects include:

- Thirst
- Mild headache
- Anxiety
- Irritability
- Aggression
- Nervousness
- Sleepiness
- Depression
- Abnormal heart rhythm
- Fainting or dizziness
- Blood clots in the legs (called deep vein thrombosis)
- Seizure
- Swollen limbs

## ANDROSTENEDIONE

Androstenedione ("andro") is a hormone produced by the adrenal glands, ovaries and testes. It's a hormone that's normally converted to testosterone and estradiol in both men and women.

---

[211] Mayo Clinic (2010) Creatine: Safety. Retrieved from http://www.mayoclinic.com/health/creatine/NS_patient-creatine/DSECTION=safety

Androstenedione is a controlled substance and its use as a performance-enhancing drug is illegal in the United States. However, it is still sold as a nutritional supplement and manufacturers and bodybuilding magazines tout its ability to allow athletes to train harder and recover more quickly.

According to Diane Hales, author of *An Invitation to Health*, scientific studies that refute these claims show that supplemental androstenedione doesn't increase testosterone and that your muscles don't get stronger with androstenedione use.[212]

*SIDE EFFECTS OF ANDROSTENEDIONE IN MEN INCLUDE:*

- Acne
- Diminished sperm production
- Shrinking of the testicles
- Enlargement of the breasts

*SIDE EFFECTS OF ANDROSTENEDIONE IN WOMEN INCLUDE:*

- Acne
- Masculinization, such as deepening of the voice and male-pattern baldness

In both men and women, androstenedione can decrease HDL cholesterol (the "good" cholesterol), which puts you at greater risk of heart attack and stroke.

---

[212] Hales, D. (2008) *An Invitation to Health*. Brookes/Cole: Independence, KY

## Stimulants

Some athletes use stimulants for the perceived edge they give in stimulating the central nervous system and increasing heart rate and blood pressure.

Stimulants can:

- Reduce fatigue
- Suppress appetite
- Increase alertness and aggressiveness

Common stimulants include:

- Caffeine and amphetamines (Dexedrine, Adderall)
- Street drugs such as cocaine and methamphetamine
- Cold remedies, which often contain the stimulants ephedrine or pseudoephedrine hydrochloride (Sudafed, Advil Allergy Sinus)

Although stimulants can boost physical performance and promote aggressiveness on the field, their side effects can also impair athletic performance.

- Nervousness and irritability make it hard to concentrate on the game.
- Insomnia can prevent an athlete from getting needed sleep.
- Athletes may become psychologically addicted or develop a tolerance so that they need greater amounts to achieve the desired effect, meaning they'll take doses

that are much higher than the intended medical dose.

Other side effects include:

- Heart palpitations
- Heart rhythm abnormalities
- Weight loss
- Tremors
- Mild hypertension
- Hallucinations
- Convulsions
- Heart attack and other circulatory problems

# DHEA

DHEA (dehydroepiandrosterone) is one of the hormones produced by the adrenal glands. After being secreted by the adrenal glands, it circulates in the bloodstream as DHEA-sulfate (DHEAS) and is converted as needed into other hormones.[213]

A synthetic form of this hormone is available as a supplement in tablet, capsule, liquid, and sublingual form. Some products claim to contain "natural" DHEA precursors from wild yam. However, the body cannot convert these substances into DHEA.

---

[213] The NIH National Library of Medicine — Dehydroepiandrosterone http://www.nlm.nih.gov/medlineplus/druginfo/natural/patient-dhea.html

Some athletes believe that DHEA promotes the loss of body fat and since it is a precursor to testosterone, DHEA may help build muscle mass. [214]

Several studies have shown DHEA use may increase the risks of prostate cancer in men and endometrial cancer in women. Medical experts suggest that before taking DHEA supplements, individuals should have a blood test to determine existing DHEA and other hormone (testosterone or estrogen) levels.

DHEA should not be taken by men who have a history of prostate problems or by women with a history of breast, ovarian, or uterine cancer. It is not recommended for anyone under age 40, or by women who are pregnant, nursing, or who can still bear children. Women who are taking an estrogen replacement, who have a history of heart disease, and anyone with other significant health problems should consult their doctor before taking DHEA.

Men taking DHEA should have regular PSA tests and women should have periodic mammograms, because DHEA may promote the growth of breast cancer.[215]

## SIDE EFFECTS

Some side effects have been reported and are usually associated with doses of 5 mg a day or more. These

---

[214] Calfee, R.; Fadale, P. (March 2006). "Popular ergogenic drugs and supplements in young athletes". *Pediatrics* 117 (3): e577–89. doi:10.1542/peds.2005-1429.

[215] Tworoger, S. S.; Missmer, S. A.; Eliassen, A. H. *et al.* (2006). "The association of plasma DHEA and DHEA sulfate with breast cancer risk in predominantly premenopausal women". *Cancer Epidemiol. Biomarkers Prev.* 15 (5): 967–71. doi:10.1158/1055-9965.EPI-05-0976.

include acne, body and facial hair growth in women, enlarged breasts in men, scalp hair loss, anxiety, insomnia, headaches, mood changes, and fatigue. It can cause menstrual irregularities in women under age 50, and may decrease HDL (good cholesterol) in women. A few cases of irregular heart rhythm have been reported in people taking 25-50 mg a day of DHEA.[216],[217]

Although long-term safety data on DHEA does not exist, side effects at high intakes (50–200 mg per day) appear to include:

- Acne (in over 50% of people)
- Increased facial hair (18%)
- Increased perspiration (8%)

In a preliminary trial, DHEA was also reported to induce less common side effects, including:

- Breast tenderness
- Weight gain
- Mood alteration
- Headache
- Oily skin and
- Menstrual irregularity in some women.

Since this trial was not controlled, some of these less common "side effects" might have occurred even with a

---

[216] Tokish, J. M.; Kocher, M. S.; Hawkins, R. J. (2004). "Ergogenic aids: a review of basic science, performance, side effects, and status in sports". *The American Journal of Sports Medicine* 32 (6): 1543–53. doi:10.1177/0363546504268041

[217] Medline Plus. "DHEA". *Drugs and Supplements Information*. National Library of Medicine. http://www.nlm.nih.gov/medlineplus/druginfo/natural/patient-dhea.html#Safety. Retrieved 18 February 2010.

placebo. A case of mania was reported in an older man who took 200–300 mg of DHEA per day for six months. However, in that case report, other causes of mania could not be ruled out.

Significant increases in testosterone levels in both men and women have been reported in some trials. Other reports have found this change in women but not in men. An increase in testosterone may increase the risk of several cancers, and high amounts of DHEA have caused cancer in animals. According to The American Cancer Society, "Caution is advised in their use [DHEA] in people who have cancer, especially types of cancer that respond to hormones, such as certain types of breast cancer, prostate cancer, and uterine cancer. People younger than 30 may run the risk of suppressing the body's natural production of DHEA if they take DHEA supplements." While there are hints that DHEA may have some use in treating certain hormone deficiencies, autoimmune diseases, and mood and memory problems of older age, more research is needed to determine its long-term safety and effectiveness.[218]

## NON-DRUG ALTERNATIVES

The promise of a wonder drug that makes you an athletic star overnight is obviously appealing. But for those that are looking for a permanent, positive change, drugs are seldom the answer. And as we have seen in

---

[218] The American Cancer Society (2013) DHEA .
http://www.cancer.org/treatment/treatmentsandsideeffects/comple
mentaryandalternativemedicine/pharmacologicalandbiologicaltreatme
nt/dhea

this chapter, they can cause more problems than they cure.

Although I co-own a company that uses non-drug approaches for Peak Performance, I can say that my opinion on this matter is not based on financials. It is based upon our results with the people who walk through our door every day. Many of our

patients come to us seeking a safe way to improve their athletic performance. Others have tried medications that did not cure the underlying cause of the problem, and were then struggling with the medications' effects, or they find they were unable to discontinue the medication without significant withdrawal symptoms.

Permanent improvement without drugs requires a willingness on the part of the patients to complete the training regimen and a desire to make permanent change. Those who qualify for our training experience found a new ability to exert control over their own bodies and a whole new outlook on life.

We are gratified by the success of our patients/clients. We cannot guarantee success, of course, but the results we have seen demonstrate that the training we provide is effective and helps our patients/clients live better lives.

# CHAPTER 7
# FEEDING THE BRAIN

The American diet has changed dramatically since the early part of the twentieth century. Our diets once consisted of locally grown and raised foodstuffs with natural preservatives (if any) and flavorings such as sugar and salt. This relatively benign diet has been replaced with one filled with fast food and empty calories, an excess of corn-based sugars, synthetic flavorings, artificial colorings, saturated fats and genetically modified and chemically altered foods.

These changes occurred incrementally. Each new development had a specific purpose—to stave off decay or to improve flavor and color. Some were merely to improve shelf life or to present a more pleasing appearance in the store or on the plate. But taken as a whole, these changes have wrought profound changes in the quality and quantity of the food in our diets.

We are seeing the effects of these changes in our bodies, as well. Obesity, cancer, heart disease, stroke and intestinal disorders are skyrocketing and hormone imbalances are becoming much more apparent in our society.

Although we recently "reformed" the healthcare system in America, little was said about reforming the food system. It is time to monitor our own food and to take note of the effects on our health. Michael Pollan, author of *The Omnivore's Dilemma*, wrote in the New York Times, "The American way of eating has become the elephant in the room in the debate over health care ... The health care industry finds it more profitable to treat chronic diseases than to prevent them."

Although research on how food affects the brain and behavior is relatively new, we now know that particular nutrients alter brain chemistry, causing changes in brain function, mood and behavior. The truth is that what we eat has a direct effect on the production of chemical signals in the brain.[219]

Even our water has been affected. In the last few years we've seen a huge increase in pharmaceuticals measured in public water supplies.[220] This issue is just now receiving more public attention, but with the rise in pharmaceutical consumption, their metabolites and unmetabolized excesses are flushed from our bodies through our feces and urine. Then we flush this drug-rich waste into our sewer systems.

The water purification systems used by municipalities were never designed to remove medical products from the waste water. Thus, the drug residues are released into the groundwater and find their way back into the public drinking water. The result is that we inadvertently ingest small doses of many unprescribed drugs every time we consume public water.

---

[219] New York Times (1979) Chemical curbs memory losses,. January 9, 1979, Part 3, pp. 1; 5.
[220] National Institute of Environmental Health Sciences (2005) Damming the Flow of Drugs into Drinking Water. *Environmental Health Perspectives*, Oct. 2005, *13*, 10.

Let's look at some specific components of our diets and how they relate to our bodily environment.

## SUGAR

Sugar is a simple carbohydrate found naturally in many foods, including fruits and grains. However, refined sugar contains no fiber, minerals, proteins, fats or enzymes, and provides only empty calories.[221]

Dr. Gary Farr describes the process of refining sugar as follows, "In the repeated processes of washing, boiling, centrifuging, filtering and drying, nearly all of the plant's nutritional elements are lost. What remains in the raw sugar product is 95% sucrose along with nutritionally insignificant minerals." *Raw Sugar* is not a raw or natural product at all, but is the highly refined, nutritionally depleted, 95% sucrose product before it is even further refined. Sucrose in its completely refined stage is more familiarly called table sugar.

If sanitized by steaming, this "raw sugar" can be marketed as *turbinado*. To produce the white crystals we call table sugar, bleaching agents such as lime and carbon dioxide are added. The sugar is then "purified" (refined) further and whitened by filtration, thus removing even more minerals. ("Pure" sugar refers to chemical purity, devoid of all nutritional and other elements, and not to a wholesome quality.)

Over 99.9% of the completely refined white sugar product we now buy is sucrose, which for all practical

---

[221] Greenly, L.W. (2007) A Doctor's Guide to Diet Plans from A-Z. *Journal of Chiropractic Medicine, 3* (1), 25-32. doi:10.1016/S0899-3467(07)60064-0

purposes contains no nutritional elements such as vitamins, minerals, proteins or fiber.

What happens when you eat a refined carbohydrate like sugar? Your body must borrow vital nutrients from healthy cells to metabolize the incomplete food. Calcium, sodium, potassium and magnesium are taken from various parts of the body to make use of the sugar. Often so much calcium is used to neutralize the effects of sugar that the bones become brittle. The withdrawn calcium and ultimately compromises immune function.[222] Because sugar is devoid of minerals, vitamins, fiber, and has such a deteriorating effect on the endocrine system, researchers and major health organizations (American Dietetic Association and American Diabetic Association) agree that sugar consumption in America is one of the three major causes of degenerative disease.

We've known since 1931 that cancer cells crave sugar; excess sugar feeds rapidly dividing cancer cells. Otto Warburg, Ph.D., a German researcher was given the Nobel Prize in Medicine for his discovery that cancer cells depend mainly on glucose for their food supply.[223]

Cancer cells devour glucose without the aid of oxygen. This produces a large buildup of lactic acid which in turn creates a more acidic pH in and around cancerous tissues. An acidic pH in the body contributes to the overall physical fatigue experienced by cancer patients.

---

[222] Dean, C. (2009) The Scary Truth About Sugar. Retrieved from: http://www.carolyndean.com/articles_scary_truth_about_sugar.html
[223] Feldman, B. (2000) The Nobel Prize: A History of Genius, Controversy and Prestige. New York: Arcade Publishing.

There have been numerous studies in peer-reviewed journals show that sugar increases prostate, colon, and biliary tract cancer.[224]

Today sugar is being sold in several forms:

- Sucrose (table sugar)
- Dextrose (corn sugar)
- High-fructose corn syrup (which is processed into many common foods such as bread, breakfast cereal, mayonnaise, peanut butter, ketchup and spaghetti sauce)

In the last 20 years, we have increased sugar consumption in the U.S. dramatically.[225] Before the end of the 19th century it was estimated that an individual consumed five pounds of sugar per year. Today the estimated consumption of sugar per individual has grown to 135 pounds per year![226]

According to Marion Nestle, chair of the Department of Nutrition and Food Studies at New York University, "Because sugary foods often replace more healthful foods, diets high in sugar are almost certainly contributing to osteoporosis, cancer, and heart disease."[227] Sugar also raises the body's insulin level

---

[224] Krebs, H.A. (1972) Otto Heinrich Warburg. 1883-1970. Biographical Memoirs of Fellows of the Royal Society. *The Royal Society, 18,* 628–699. doi:10.1098/rsbm.1972.0023.

[225] Steenhuysen, J. (2010) U.S. heart group draws hard line on sugar I take. Reuters. Retrieved from: http://www.reuters.com/article/idUSN24165384

[226] Volk T, et al. (1993) pH in human tumor xenografts: effect of intravenous administration of glucose. Br J *Cancer, 68*(3), 492-500.

[227] Nestle, M. (1988) Surgeon General's Report on Diet and Health

which inhibits the release of growth hormones, depressing the immune system.

In the last 30 years, researchers have also found a connection between consumption of sugar and vitamin C. Vitamin C is used by white blood cells to *phagocytize*, or engulf and destroy, bacteria or other foreign materials. White blood cells require a 50-times higher concentration of Vitamin C inside the cell than outside in order to function optimally. [228]

Glucose and Vitamin C have similar chemical structures, so that if sugar levels rise, less vitamin C allowed into cells. It takes very little; a blood sugar value of 120 reduces the phagocytic index by 75%. Thus, when you eat sugar, your immune system is significantly challenged.[229]

Simple sugars have been observed to aggravate asthma, mood swings, personality changes, mental illness, nervous disorders, diabetes, heart disease, gallstones, hypertension, and arthritis.[230]

John Hoebel, a psychologist at Princeton University in New Jersey, conducted research on whether it is possible to become dependent upon large amounts of

---

[228] Digirolamo, M. (1994) Diet and cancer: markers, prevention and treatment. New York: Plenum Press.
[229] Simon, J. A. & Hudes, E. S. (1999) Serum ascorbic acid and other correlates of self-reported cataract among older Americans. *J Clin Epidemiol.*, *52*(12), 1207-1211.
[230] American Society of Clinical Oncology (2000) Annual meeting, New Orleans, May 23PMID: 16059792

sugar.[231] Together with a team of physiologists from the University of the Andes in Merida, Venezuela, Hoebel showed that rats fed a diet containing 25% sugar suffer high anxiety when the sugar is removed. Symptoms included chattering teeth and the shakes—similar, he says, to those seen in people withdrawing from nicotine or morphine.

When naloxone, a drug that blocks opioid receptors was given to the rats, a drop in dopamine levels in the nucleus accumbens was observed, as well as an increase in acetylcholine release. (The nucleus accumbens is an area in the brain involved in motivation and reward to feeding and drug addiction.) This is the same neurochemical pattern found in heroin addicts as they go into opioid withdrawal. [232]

"The implication is that some animals—and by extension some people—can become overly dependent on sweet food," says Hoebel. "The brain is getting addicted to its own opioids as it would morphine or heroin. Drugs give a bigger effect, but it's essentially the same process." It is also good to remember that sugars are carbohydrates. Dietary carbohydrates also include the complex carbohydrates, starch and fiber. During digestion all carbohydrates except fiber break down into sugars.[233]

---

[231] Avena, N. M., Rada, P., Hoebel, B. G. (2010) Evidence for sugar addiction: Behavioral and neurochemical effects of intermittent, excessive sugar intake. *Neurosci & Biobehav Rev, 32* (1), 20-39.

[232] Carlo Calantuoni et al(2002) Evidence That Intermittent, Excessive Sugar Intake Causes Endogenous Opioid Dependence, *Obesity Research*, Volume 10, Number 6, pp. 478-488, June 2002.

[233] BBC News (2003) Fast Food as Addictive as Heroin. Retrieved from: http://news.bbc.co.uk/2/hi/health/2707143.stm

*SUGAR SUBSTITUTES*

The effects of sugar in diets have been well documented. In order to reduce sugars in their diet, many people use sugar substitutes or artificial sweeteners. The substitutes are added to foods to make food taste sweet without the calories. In the United States, sweeteners fall under the Generally Recognized as Safe (GRAS) list or as food additives under the 1958 Food Additives Amendment to the Federal Food, Drug, and Cosmetic Act.

There are two general classes of sweeteners, nutritive and non-nutritive. Nutritive sweeteners contain calories and provide energy, while non-nutritive sweeteners have no calories and provide no energy.

## Non-Nutritive Sweeteners

High intensity, non-nutritive (zero calories per serving) sugar substitutes include aspartame, acesulfame-K, saccharin and sucralose.

- Aspartame—(NutraSweet®, Equal®) Discovered in 1965, currently more than half the adult American population consumes products containing aspartame. A multibillion-dollar industry aggressively promotes thousands of items containing this chemical sweetener that consumers use in large amounts to avoid sugar or lose weight. There is mounting evidence that aspartame causes or aggravates headache, seizures, depression, many neurologic disorders (most notably multiple sclerosis), visual difficulty, allergies, diabetic complications, as well as a host of other conditions. It has also been reported that aspartame has the potential for addiction.[234] It is made from a combination of the two amino acids, aspartic acid and phenylalanine. During digestion, aspartame is broken down into these two individual amino acids. It is also broken down when exposed to heat, resulting in a loss of its sweet taste. Aspartame is 160-220 times sweeter than sucrose. In fact, it has the same calories as sugar, but since it is so sweet and such a small amount is needed for the sweetening effect, it is labeled as zero calories per serving.

- Acesulfame-K — acesulfame potassium, (Sunette, Sweet One®, Sweet 'n Safe) Discovered in 1967, acesulfame-K is 150-200 times sweeter than sugar and commonly used as a tabletop sweetener. Acesulfame-K is the result of the combination of acetoacetic acid and potassium to form a highly stable, crystalline sweetener. The chemical structure is similar to saccharin.

Acesulfame-K is usually used in combination with aspartame or other sweeteners because it enhances and sustains the sweet taste of foods and beverages and helps extend the shelf life of food product it is in. It is heat stable which means that it can be used in baked products.

It does not provide calories since the body does not metabolize it; it is excreted in the urine without change. According to Michael F. Jacobeson, Ph.D., author of Safe Food, "Even compared to aspartame and saccharin (which are afflicted with their own safety problems), acesulfame K is the worst. The

---

[234] Roberts, HJ (2000) Aspartame, (NutraSweet) Addiction. http://www.dorway.com/tldaddic.html

additive is inadequately tested; the FDA based its approval on tests which were short of their own standards of acesulfame K. But even those tests indicate that the additive can cause cancer in animals, which means it may increase cancer risk in humans. In l987, CSPI urged the FDA not to approve acesulfame K, but was ignored. After the FDA gave the chemical its blessing, CSPI urged that it be banned. The FDA hasn't yet ruled on that request."

Acesulfame-K can be found in about 4,000 foods, including chewing gum, desserts, alcoholic beverages, syrups, candies, sauces, and yogurt. In the US it is found in Hershey's Lite Syrup® and Fat Free Dutch Chocolate Hot Cocoa, Trident® chewing gum and sugar-free Jell-O®.

- Saccharin — (Sweet'N Low®, Sugar Twin®)
Saccharin was discovered at Johns Hopkins in 1879 and is estimated to be 200-700 times sweeter than sugar. It is calorie-free because the body cannot break it down.

In 1977, after a study found it caused bladder cancer in rats, all products that contained saccharin were required to be labeled with the following statement: "Use of this product may be hazardous to your health. This product contains saccharin which has been determined to cause cancer in laboratory animals."

Studies have followed diabetics who have used saccharin for years and have yet to show an increase in the incidence of bladder cancer. On May 15, 2000 the U.S. government released a report on things known to cause cancer. When the list came out, it "de-listed" saccharin from the list of suspected carcinogens. Even if you don't use the "pink packets," you likely are still consuming saccharin. It is found in non-food products such as Listerine®, Crest® Toothpaste, Robitussin® cough syrup, and Carefree® chewing gum. It is also in salad dressings, jam, jelly, preserves and baked goods.

- Sucralose — (Splenda®) Sucralose was discovered in 1976 by British scientists looking for a new pesticide. Sucralose is 600 times sweeter than sugar and is made from chlorinated sugar. The molecular structure of the molecule, however, is closer to a pesticide than a sugar. There has been very little research done on the effects of sucralose, however evidence that there are side effects of Splenda is accumulating little by little. For example, sucralose has been implicated as a possible migraine trigger. Self-reported adverse reactions to Splenda or sucralose collected by the Sucralose Toxicity Information Center include skin rashes/flushing, panic-like agitation, dizziness and numbness, diarrhea, swelling, muscle aches, headaches, intestinal cramping, bladder issues, and stomach pain. These show up at one end of the spectrum — in the people who have an allergy or sensitivity to the sucralose molecule. But there is no evidence how Splenda consumption affects the rest of us; there are no long-term studies in humans with large numbers of subjects to say if it's safe for everyone.[235]

---

[235] Pick, M. (2005) Sugar substitutes and the potential danger of Splenda. Retrieved from:
http://www.womentowomen.com/healthyweight/splenda.aspx

## HIGH FRUCTOSE CORN SYRUP

Today, we are not only eating much more sugar in our diet than ever before, we are also consuming sugar that we don't even realize is there. One of the reasons is the widespread use of High Fructose Corn Syrup or *HFCS*, in everything from bread to mayonnaise. High fructose corn syrup also masquerades under the name crystalline fructose in Glaceau Vitamin Water and some energy drinks.

HFCS has been at the center of health and industry debates for years. The HFCS industry advertises HFCS as "natural" because it's made from corn. But the truth is that HFCS does not appear in nature. HFCS is produced by converting corn starch to glucose and then to fructose to form a sweet, clear syrup. For decades, HFCS has been made using mercury grade caustic soda produced in industrial chlorine (chlor-alkali) plants.

Four years ago, the FDA had evidence that commercial HFCS was contaminated with mercury. However, the agency did not inform consumers, help change industry practices, or even conduct additional testing.[236]

It is still cheaper to manufacture HFCS than sugar because the US government subsidizes corn crops. In fact, the average US consumer pays *ten* tax dollars for

---

[236] Pusztai, A. (2002) Can Science Give Us the Tools for Recognizing Possible Health Risks for GM Food? *Nutrition and Health 16*, 73–84.

every dollar earned by Archer Daniels Midland, the largest producer of HFCS. [237]

The problem with HFCS isn't that it is costly to the consumers, but that it is many times sweeter than regular sugar and a sweeter taste sells.[238]With this in mind, it's not hard to see why food manufacturers use it so extensively. But the result is that since the 1980s when HFCS was introduced, the American obesity rates have skyrocketed, type 2 Diabetes has doubled and the number of overweight children has tripled.[239]

High fructose corn syrup is metabolized to fat in your body far more rapidly than any other sugar. HFCS blunts the body's ability to recognize when it is full and increases a person's appetite. The temporary spike of HFCS blocks the action of insulin, which typically regulates how body cells use and store sugar and other food nutrients for energy. [240] There is a rise in uric acid in the bloodstream that occurs after fructose is consumed. If uric acid levels are frequently elevated, over time features of metabolic syndrome may develop,

---

[237] Bovard, J. (1995) Archer Daniels Midland: A case study in corporate welfare, *Cato Institute*, September 26, 1995, www.cato.org/pubs/pas/pa-241.html.

[238] Philpott, T. (2005) Archer Daniels Midland's man at USDA, *Bitter Greens Journal*, April 29, 2005 http://bittergreensgazette.blogspot.com/....

[239] US Department of Health and Human Services, National Institutes of Health, (2006) National Heart, lung, and Blood Institute. Guidelines on Overweight and Obesity: Electronic Textbook. Available at: http://www.nhlbi.nih.gov/guidelines/obesity/e_txtbk/ratnl/23.htm.

[240] Sanda, B.(2003) The Double Danger of High Fructose Corn Syrup. *Wise Traditions in Food, Farming and the Healing Arts*. Weston A. Price Foundation, Winter 2003.

including high blood pressure, obesity and elevated blood cholesterol levels. [241]

Another major issue with HFCS is that it is typically manufactured using genetically modified (GM) corn. Two of the enzymes used to make the syrup, alpha amylase and glucose-isomerase, are as well.[242]

In 2009 the American Academy of Environmental Medicine called for a moratorium on GM foods and for mandatory labeling.[243] In their white paper they cited numerous animal studies that linked GM foods to adverse health effects and altered structure and function of kidneys, liver, pancreas and spleen. They also found a decrease in fertility, an increase in asthma, allergies and inflammation in those animals eating GM foods. It is also interesting to note that in animals eating GM food, they found a difference in function of 400 genes that control protein synthesis and modification, cell signaling, cholesterol synthesis and insulin regulation. [244]

Beverages made with HFCS also contain high levels of reactive carbonyls, a free radical linked to tissue

---

[241] Bray, GA; Nielsen SJ; Popkin BM (2004) "Consumption of high-fructose corn syrup in beverages may play a role in the epidemic of obesity". American Journal of Clinical Nutrition 79 (4): 537–543. PMID 15051594.

[242] Smith, J.M. (2007) Genetic Roulette: The Documented Health Risks of Genetically Engineered Foods, Yes! Books, Fairfield, IA USA 2007

[243] American Academy of Environmental Medicine (2009) Press Release for Immediate Moratorium on Genetically Modified Foods. Retrieved from: http://www.aaemonline.org/gmopressrelease.html

[244] The American Academy of Environmental Medicine (2009) Genetically Modified Foods. Retrieved from: http://www.aaemonline.org/gmopost.html

damage, diabetes and other diabetes complications. Researchers at Rutgers University found that the concentration of reactive carbonyls in a single can of soda was about 5 times the concentration found in the blood of an adult diabetic.[245]

According to Weston A. Price Foundation, HFCS also triggers a "browning" or "maillard" reaction. This reaction occurs when certain carbohydrate molecules bind with proteins and cause aging. It changes the structure of proteins and enzymes resulting in tissue and organ damage. This effect can occur with any sugar but with HFCS it happens *seven times faster* than with glucose![246]

Humans are not the only ones being affected. HFCS is also fed to bees. In 2009, researchers went looking for what has killed about one-third of the honey bees in the U.S. They found that when HFCS is heated, it forms a toxin fatal to bees called hydroxymethylfurfural (HMF).[247] Studies in Sweden have also linked HMF to DNA damage in humans.[248] In addition, HMF breaks

---

[245] American Chemical Society, (2007) press release of August 23, 2007
[246] Sandra, B. (2003) The Double Danger of High Fructose Corn Syrup, Wise Traditions, newsletter of the Weston A. Price Foundation, Winter 2003. Also H. F. Bunn & P. J. Higgins, Reaction of Nonosaccharides with roteins; Possible Evolutionary Significance, Science 213 (1981), 2222-2244.
[247] LeBlanc, B., Eggleston, G. et al. (2009) Formation of hydroxymethylfurfural in domestic high fructose corn syrup and its toxicity to the honey bee (Apis mellifera), *Journal of Agriculture and Food Science*, 57:736907376, DOI: 10.1021/jf9014526
[248] Durling, L. J., Busk, L., & Hellman, B. E. (2009) Evaluation of the DNA damaging effect of the heat-induced food toxicant 5-hydroxymethylfurfural (HMF) in various cell lines with different activities of sulfotransferases, *Food Chem Toxocology, 47* (4), 880-884.doi:10.1016/j.fct.2009.01.022

down in the body to form other substances potentially more harmful than its original form.

## GLUTEN

It is well known that gluten comprises about 80% of the protein in wheat. Less well known, however, is that gluten is used as a stabilizing agent in such diverse products as ice cream, catsup, licorice candy, imitation bacon, processed luncheon meats, soy sauce, drugs and over-the-counter medications—even communion wafers.[249]

The FDA has labeled gluten as *Generally Recognized as Safe* (GRAS), although to those with celiac disease, it can be quite unsafe. Because it is labeled as GRAS, its presence need not be disclosed on ingredient labels, a trap for the unwary [250,251]

As gluten has become more common in the foods we eat, people have been exhibiting more frequent sensitivities and allergic reactions. Reactions can include irritability, headaches, difficulty concentrating, fatigue and increased appetite. It can even produce

---

[249] Kendall, P. (2003) Gluten sensitivity more widespread than previously thought. Colorado State University Extension. Retrieved from: http://www.ext.colostate.edu/pubs/columnnn/nn030331.html.
[250] National Institutes of Health (NIH) (2004) Celiac Disease National Digestive Diseases Information Clearing House. Retrieved from: http://digestive.niddk.nih.gov/ddiseases/pubs/celiac/index.htm.
[251] National Institutes of Health (NIH) (2005) Celiac disease. Consensus Development Panel on Celiac Disease. Retrieved from: http://www.guideline.gov/summary/summary.aspx?doc_id=5692&nbr =0"http://www.guideline.gov/summary/summary.aspx?doc_id=5692& nbr=0

problems with balance resembling Multiple Sclerosis.[252]

Diagnosing sensitivity to glutens, especially in children, can be difficult, as it may appear as a seemingly disconnected list of symptoms such as attention issues, chronic earaches, stomach cramps, alternating diarrhea and constipation, bloated abdomen, joint pain, fatigue or just being small for one's age. When gluten sensitivity goes untreated, malnutrition develops, and the chronic inflammation may lead eventually to gastrointestinal cancer.[253]

Dr. Kenneth Fine, an intestinal researcher at Entero Labs, reports that as many as 40% of Americans may have the gene for gluten sensitivity. That means as many as four in ten Americans may have some delayed allergic reaction to gluten.[254]

Those involved in treating and caring for those with autism are also examining gluten and casein sensitivities. Children with autism diagnoses have shown mild to dramatic improvements in speech and/or behavior after these substances were removed from their diets. [255]

---

[252] Hadjivassiliou, M., Grünewald , R.A .et al. (1999) Gluten sensitivity: a many-headed hydra. *BMJ 1999* (318), 1710-1711.
[253] Kumar, V., Rajadhyaksha, M. et al.(2001) Celiac Disease-Associated Autoimmune Endocrinopathies. *Clin Diag Lab Immunol , 8*(4),678-685.
[254] Kharrazian, D. (2010) Why Do I Still Have Thyroid Symptoms When My Lab Tests Are Normal? New York: Morgan James Publishing.

[255] Genuis, S.J. & Bouchard, T.P. (2009) Celiac disease presenting as autism. J Child Neurol. 2010 Jan;25(1):114-9. doi: 10.1177/0883073809336127. Epub 2009 Jun 29.

---

Autism is becoming more pervasive in our society.[256] In 1997, 7-10 in 10,000 were identified as autistic, while the numbers are 1 in 100 today, according to Kathleen Sebelius, the Secretary with US Health and Human Services and the Center for Disease Control. Some speculate that the causes of autism could include genetics, environmental toxins, infectious agents, enzymatic problems, and dietary factors. Particular interest has been directed to the relation between childhood autism and problems with dairy products and the proteins that are in grain, including gluten. [257,258]

## DAIRY PRODUCTS

Milk proteins have also been identified as a major source of developmental disorders.[259]They can cause many allergic reactions, particularly in children. These proteins are found in cow's milk and its byproducts such as casein, whey, beta lactoglobin, alpha-lactoglobulin, bovine serum albumin and gamma-

---

[256] Reichelt KL, Ekrem J, Scott H. Gluten, milk proteins and autism: dietary intervention effects on behavior and peptide secretion. J Appl Nutr 1990;42:1-11.

[257] Dohan, F. C. (1983) More on celiac disease as a model for schizophrenia. *Biological Psychiatry, 18,* 561-564.

[258] Horvath, K., et al. (1999) Gastrointestinal abnormalities in children with autistic disorder. *J Pediatr. 135* (5), 559-63.

[259] Elder, J.H., Shankar, M., Shuster, J., Theriaque, D., Burns, S. & Sherrill, L. (2006) The gluten-free, casein-free diet in autism: results of a preliminary double blind clinical trial. *J Autism Dev Disord.* 2006 Apr;36(3):413-20.

lactoglobulin. Casein breaks down into casomorphine, which as implied in the name, has opioid properties. [260]

Evidence of antibodies to beta casomorphin-8 has been found in the brain stem of infants suggesting that beta-casomorphins can be transported from the blood into the brain stem.[261]

Even breast-fed infants can have problems from cow's milk previously ingested by the lactating mother.[262] Interestingly, early exposure to cow's milk in preterm infants with a family history of allergies increased their risk of developing a wide range of allergies, including eczema.[263]

Whereas intolerance to milk protein has been associated with some developmental disorders, intolerance to proteins in grain has received the most

---

[260] Jinsmaa Y, Yoshikawa M, 1999; "Enzymatic release of neocasomorphin and beta-casomorphinfrom bovine beta-casein"; *Peptides* 20:957-962

[261] Sienkiewicz-Sztapka, E., Jarmo³owska, B., Krawczuk, S., Kostyra, E. Kostyra, H. & Bielikowicz, H. (2008) Transport of bovine milk-derived opioid peptides across a Caco-2 monolayer. *International Dairy Journal. 19*(4), 252-257. doi:10.1016/j.idairyj.2008.10.007.

[262] Wilson, N. W., Self, T. W. & Hamburger, R.N. (1990) Severe cow's milk induced colitis in an exclusively breast-fed neonate. Case report and clinical review of cow's milk allergy. *Clin Pediatr (Phila) 29*(2),77-80.

[263] Lucas, A., Brooke, O.G., Morley, R., Cole, T. J.,& Bamford, M. F. (1990) Early diet of preterm infants and development of allergic or atopic disease: randomized prospective study. *BMJ. 31*(300:6728),837–840.

attention; frequently reactions to both occur in the same individual. [264], [265]

## GENETICALLY MODIFIED FOODS

The newest danger to our health and the health of our children comes from genetically modified (GM) food crops in this country. These crops are modified by artificially inserting genes from viruses, bacteria, other plant species, insects, humans, and other animals into the plant genome. This process can produce new chemicals unknown previously in our foods and animals. These genetically modified genes cause a lack of normal nutrients, while concentrating other naturally occurring plant substances until they become toxic.[266]

In 1994, a tomato was the first genetically engineered whole food product in the US. According to the Grocery Manufacturer Association, since then 75-80 % of all processed foods in U.S. grocery stores now contain ingredients from genetically modified organisms. [267] Corn, soybeans and cotton— the number 1, 2 and 5

[264] Lahey, M. & Rosen, S. (2013) Developmental Disorders And Dairy Products, Grains, Gluten And Other Proteins. Retrieved from: http://www.childrensdisabilities.info/allergies/developmentaldisorder sprotein7.html

[265] Ortolani. C. & Pastorello, E.A. (2006) Food allergies and food intolerances. *Best Pract Res Clin Gastroenterol* 20 (3): 467–83. doi:10.1016/j.bpg.2005.11.010

[266] Smith, J.M. (2007) Genetic Roulette: The Documented Health Risks of Genetically Engineered Foods, Fairfield, IA: Yes! Books.

[267] Gurian-Sherman, D. (2012) Genetically Engineered Food: An Overview (Food & Water Watch, 2012) Retrieved from: http://www.ucsusa.org/assets/documents/food_and_agriculture/failu re-to-yield.pdf

crops in America, respectively,—are the country's top genetically modified harvests. [23]

In 1996, only 2.2 % of U.S. acres growing corn featured gene-spliced varieties; Today, GM crops have taken over 85-91% (nearly 171 million acres) of US planting of the three crops listed in the previous paragraph.[268]

## SOME OF THE RISKS

A number of unanswered issues with GM crops are surfacing. According to Artemis Dona and Ioannis S. Arvanitoyannis in their article "Health Risks of Genetically Modified Foods," the majority of the rather few studies conducted with GM foods, indicate that they may cause hepatic, pancreatic, renal, and reproductive effects and may alter hematological, biochemical, and immunologic parameters the significance of which remains unknown. [269] These results indicate that many GM foods have some common toxic effects. Thus, further studies should be conducted in order to explore the mechanisms causing these effects.

Small amounts of ingested DNA may not be broken down by digestive processes and there is a possibility that this DNA may either enter the bloodstream or be excreted, especially in individuals with abnormal

---

[268] Institute of Science in Society (2009) GM Crops Facing Meltdown in the US. Retrieved from: http://www.i-sis.org.uk/GMCropsFacingMeltdown.php
[269] Dona, A. & Arvanitoyannis, I. S. (2009) Health Risks of Genetically Modified Foods. Critical Reviews in Food Science and Nutrition, 49 (2), 164 – 175.

---

digestion as a result of chronic gastrointestinal disease or with immunodeficiency. [270]

Bt (*Bacillus thuringiensis*) is an insecticidal poison that is present in most genetically engineered U.S. crops that are part of animal feed and pet foods. High levels of Bt toxin in GM crops have made farmers ill and poisoned farm animals eating crop residues. [271] Bt has also been linked to autism.[272]

Bt toxin also harms microorganisms in the soil that are vital to plant health. High levels are created when GM crop residues are mulched or ploughed into the soil. [273]

Genetic material in GM herbicide-resistant soybeans can be transferred to bacteria in our digestive systems. This means that foreign proteins could be

---

[270] Horvath, K., et al. (1999) Gastrointestinal abnormalities in children with autistic disorder. *J Pediatr*. *135* (5), 559-63.

[271] Benbrook,C. (2004) Genetically Engineered Crops and Pesticide Use in the United States: The First Nine Years; BioTech InfoNet, Technical Paper Number 7. October 2004 -

[272] LaLama, A. (2009) Reversing Autism: Connecting the pieces with the latest research on Bt, Hg, Octopamine, Succinic acid, B12, Leptu and BIRM. Retrieved from: http://www.autismone.com/content/reversing-autism-connecting-pieces-latest-research-bthg-octopamine-succinic-acid-b12-leptu-

[273] Domingo, J.L. "Toxicity Studies of Genetically Modified Plants: A Review of the Published Literature." Critical Reviews in Food Science and Nutrition, 47(8):721"733. 2007.

manufactured in our own digestive systems by such bacteria, turning them into pesticide factories. [274]

So called "overexpression" can occur when spliced genes that manufacture chemicals such as Bt become hyperactive inside the plant and result in potentially toxic plant tissues. These are lethal not just to mealworms and other crop pests, but also to, birds, butterflies, other wildlife, and possibly to humans and their pets.[275]

*Glufosinate* and *glyphosate* are herbicides that are liberally applied across the U.S. and in many other countries to millions of acres of crops which have been genetically engineered to be resistant to these herbicides. These poisons are actually absorbed by the crops, while all else growing in the fields and much of the surrounding aquatic life in rivers and lakes are wiped out. The result has also produced herbicide-resistant weeds, constituting a new phenomenon of intensification; the "transgenic treadmill".[276]

These widely used herbicides have caused kidney damage and other health problems in animals. They

---

[274] Dona, A., & Arvanitoyannis, I. (2009) Health risks of genetically modified foods. *Critical Reviews in Food Science and Nutrition.* 49: 164-175. 2009.

[275] Fox, M. W. (2009) Genetic Engineering and Cloning in Animal Agriculture: Bioethical and Food Safety Concerns. Paper presented at International Conference on Sustainable Agriculture, Opatija, Croatia. Retrieved from: http://www.twobitdog.com/drfox/Animal-Cloning-Genetic-Engineering

[276] Binimelis, R., Pengue, W. & Monterros, I. (2009) "Transgenic treadmill": Responses to the emergence and spread of glyphosate-resistant johnsongrass in Argentina. *Geoforum, 40,* (4),623-633.

can cause endocrine disruption and birth defects in frogs and is lethal to many amphibians. Glyphosate has been linked with non-Hodgkin lymphoma, miscarriages and premature births in humans.[277]

These herbicides and other agrichemicals, including the insecticide Bt, are found in pet foods and the crops and crop by-products fed to cattle, pigs, poultry, and dairy cows.[278]

Many nutritionists and health experts are linking the rise in human food allergies—skin problems and inflammatory/irritable bowel syndromes—to the increased consumption of GM foods and food additives, especially genetically engineered soy products that contain novel proteins. The high incidence of skin and food allergies and other suspected allergies associated with digestive disorders and inflammatory bowel disease in dogs and cats may well be caused or aggravated by these novel proteins and other chemical contaminants in GM crop byproducts.[279], [280]

---

[277] Pusztai, A., Bardocz, S., & Ewen, S.W.B. (2003) Genetically Modified Foods: Potential Human Health Effects. Mello, J.P.F., ed., Food Safety: Contaminants and Toxins, pp. 347-372, CAB International, Wallingford Oxon, UK.

[278] Center for Disease Control (2009) Fourth Annual Report on Human Exposure to Environmental Chemicals. Retrieved from: http://www.cdc.gov/exposurereport/?id=77&tid=20"http://www.cdc.gov/exposur ereport/?id=77&tid=20

[279] Fox, M. W. (2009b) Genetic Engineering and Cloning in Animal Agriculture: Bioethical and Food Safety Concerns. Paper presented at International Conference on Sustainable Agriculture, Opatija, Croatia. Retrieved from: http://www.twobitdog.com/drfox/Animal-Cloning-Genetic-Engineering

Although there is no confirmed link, it is likely not just a coincidence that in October 2008, the US Centers for Disease Control and Prevention reported an 18% increase in allergies in children under the age of 18 between the years 1997 and 2007. Some three million children now suffer from food or digestive allergies with symptoms including vomiting, skin rashes, and breathing problems. These children take longer to outgrow milk and egg allergies and show a doubling of adverse reactions to peanuts.[281]

Adverse or unexplained effects of GM foods have occurred in almost every study on animals, including inflammation and abnormal cell growth (possibly pre-cancerous) in the stomach and small intestines, abnormal development, inflammation, and cellular changes in the liver, kidney, testicles, heart, pancreas, brain, and poor growth and above-normal mortalities.[282,283]

---

[280] Boyd, et al. (1990) Behavioural and neurochemical changes associated with chronic exposure to low level concentrations of pesticide mixtures, *Journal of Toxicology and Environmental Health*, *30*, 209 - 221.

[281] Center for Disease Control (2009) Prevalence of Autism Spectrum Disorders-Autism and Developmental Disabilities Monitoring Network, United States, 2006. *Morbidity and Mortality Weekly Report, 2009* (58), SS-10.

[282] Velimirov A., Binter, C., & Zentek, J. (2008) Biological effects of transgenic maize NK603xMON810 fed in long term reproduction studies in mice. *Report, Forschungsberichte der Sektion IV*, Band 3. Institut für Ernährung, and Forschungsinttitut für biologischen Landbau, Vienna, Austria, November 2008

[283] Fox, M. W. (2009) Conflicts of Interest in the Veterinary Profession and the Origin of Man-Made Dog and Cat Diseases. Retrieved from: http://advocacy.britannica.com/blog/advocacy/2009/07/conflicts-of-interest-in-theveterinary-profession/

Unlike conventionally bred crops, researchers found GM varieties are intrinsically unstable and prone to spontaneous mutations. These mutations make it difficult to know if what is being grown, harvested, processed, and consumed is really safe and nutritious. [284]

The inserted genes can also have unforeseen consequences, the so-called multiple pleiotropic effects.[285] Introducing a new genetic trait or quality often has unintended consequences which can include alterations in existing gene function and interrelationships with other genes. A dramatic example of this is occurred in the genetically engineered pigs that were created at the U.S. government's research facility in Beltsville, Maryland to carry human growth genes. Multiple health problems occurred including, crippling arthritis and bone-growth deformities. The genetically altered pigs also had impaired immune and reproductive systems. [286]

Multiple pleiotropic effects in GM soy include excesses of certain phytoestrogens, and the presence of anti-

---

[284] Malatesta, M., et al. (2008) Hepatoma tissue culture (HTC) cells as a model for investigating the effects of low concentrations of herbicide on cell structure and function. *Toxicology in Vitro, 22*(8), 1853-1860.
[285] Baldassarre, H., Schirm, M., Deslauriers, J., Turcotte, C. & Bordignon, V. (2009) Protein profile and alpha-lactalbumin concentration in the milk of standard and transgenic goats expressing recombinant human butyrylcholinesterase. *Transgenic Res. 18*(4), 621-632.

[286] Fox, M.W., Hodgkins, E., & Smart, M. (2009) Not Fit For A Dog: The Truth About Manufactured Dog and Cat Food. Sanger, Calif., Quill Driver Books.

---

nutrient substances, some of which could be a consequence of genomic interaction with mutagenic agrichemicals compounded by the poor nutrition (and nutritive value) of conventionally grown, rather than organically grown, crops.[287]

Herbicide food residues, combined with the unknown consequences by transgenic DNA segments (from the genes of all GM foods) becoming incorporated into the bacterial DNA can disrupt the delicate bacterial balance in the digestive system.[288] Dr. Jennifer Armstrong, President of The American Academy of Environmental Medicine (AAEM), says, "Physicians are probably seeing the effects in their patients, but need to know how to ask the right questions."

World renowned biologist Pushpa M. Bhargava goes one step further. After reviewing more than 600 scientific journals, he concludes that genetically modified organisms (GMOs) are a major contributor to the sharply deteriorating health of Americans. [289]

Biologist David Schubert of the Salk Institute warns that "...children are the most likely to be adversely effected by toxins and other dietary problems..."

[287] Fox, M. W. (2009b) Genetic Engineering and Cloning in Animal Agriculture: Bioethical and Food Safety Concerns. Paper presented at International Conference on Sustainable Agriculture, Opatija, Croatia. Retrieved from: ttp://www.twobitdog.com/drfox/Animal-Cloning-Genetic-Engineering

[288] Finamore, A., Roselli, M., Britti, S., et al. (2008) Intestinal and peripheral immune response to MON 810 maize ingestion in weaning and old mice. *J Agric. Food Chem. 56* (23), 11533-11539.

[289] Bhargava, P. M. & Suresh, N. (2009) Editorial: Biotech in India — History, present and promises. Biotechnology Journal, 4 ( 3), 286 – 287.

related to GM foods. He says that "...without adequate studies, children become the experimental animals." [290]

In one experiment, when GM soy was fed to female rats, most of their babies died within three weeks, compared to a 10% death rate among the control group fed natural soy. The GM-fed babies were also smaller and later had problems getting pregnant. When male rats were fed GM soy, their testicles actually changed color—from the normal pink to dark blue. Also, mice fed GM soy had altered young sperm.[291]

In the United States, about two dozen farmers reported thousands of pigs became sterile after consuming certain GM corn varieties. Some had false pregnancies; others gave birth to bags of water. Cows and bulls also became infertile when fed the same corn. In the US human population, the incidence of low birth weight babies, infertility, and infant mortality have all been escalating.[292] Whether this is the result of the consumption of GM food or not has not been established, however.

GM corn and cotton are engineered to produce an internal pesticide in every cell. Genetic engineers insert Bt genes into corn and cotton, so that the plants do the

---

[290] Schubert, D. (2009) A different perspective on GM food. *Nature Biotechnology, 20* , 969.

[291] Finamore, A., Roselli, M., Britti, S., et al. (2008) Intestinal and peripheral immune response to MON 810 maize ingestion in weaning and old mice. J Agric. Food Chem. 56 (23), 11533-11539.

[292] Kues ,W.A., Schwinzer, R., Wirth, D., Verhoeyen, E., Lemme, E., Herrmann, D . et al. (2006) Epigenetic silencing and tissue independent expression of a novel tetracycline inducible system in double-transgenic pigs. *FASEB J. 20*(8), 1200-1202.

killing. When bugs bite the plant, the poison splits open their stomach and kills them.[293]

The gene inserted into GM soy also transfers into the DNA of bacteria living inside our intestines and continues to function, according to a 2004 study in Nature Biotechnology. This means that eating a corn chip produced from Bt corn might transform our intestinal bacteria into living pesticide factories, possibly for the rest of our lives.[294]

No U.S. government safety studies are required on GMOs. It is up to Monsanto and the other biotech companies to determine if their foods are safe.[295] The American Academy of Environmental Medicine (AAEM) has called for a moratorium on GMO foods, in lieu of waiting another decade or two for what we see in animal studies to show up in human experience.[296]

It is a good call. Jeffrey Smith, author of Genetic Roulette [297] says,

---

[293] World Health Organization (2002) Foods derived from modern technology: 20 questions on genetically modified foods. Available from:
http://www.who.int/foodsafety/publications/biotech/20questions/en/index.html

[294] Gómez-Barbero, M., Berbel, J. & Rodríguez-Cerezo, E. (2004) Bt corn in Spain—the performance of the EU's first GM crop. Nature Biotechnology 26, 384 – 386. doi:10.1038/nbt0408-384

[295] Domingo, J. L. (2000) Health risks of genetically modified foods: Many opinions but few data. Science 288, 1748-1749

[296] American Academy of Environmental Medicine (2009) Press Release for Immediate Moratorium on Genetically Modified Foods. Retrieved from: http://www.aaemonline.org/gmopressrelease.html

[297] Smith, J.M. (2007) Genetic Roulette: The Documented Health Risks of Genetically Engineered Foods, Fairfield, IA: Yes! Books.

---

*"Many of the top researchers at the FDA know how dangerous GM food is but they are not permitted to say anything so, officially, the FDA does nothing to warn us about the potential for serious harm.*

*"Food can help introduce antibiotic resistance and it also carries a virus than can lead to the development of various 'stealth infections' which may not be detected on today's standard tests for infections. This means that although we are all focused on things like lead or mercury or food sensitivities, even the most astute doctors are doing little to combat the ever-present infection component contributing to our current health crisis."*

At the Second Annual Lyme-Autism Connection Conference held in June, 2008 in Palm Springs, discussion focused on Lyme-induced autism (LIA). Andrea Lalama, parent of an autistic boy received a standing ovation for her investigation into the Bt pesticide found in all GM corn and how it contributes to autism. She initially believed her son contracted autism after receiving 5 vaccines in one day. However, even though she found the vaccines worsened her son's speech delay problem, turning it into a case of extreme autism, she came to see a link between autism and Bt. "During WWII, Bt spores were looked at by the Germans," she reported. "They saw crystals inside the spores that puncture the intestine of the insect and give it Leaky Gut. The bacteria then get out of the intestine. The crystals keep the holes in the intestine from ever growing back together again and healing."

Bt has been used as a spray pesticide in the USA since 1939. Autism first appeared in 1943. "The Bt pesticide was introduced into genetically modified corn, then potatoes, then fruits and vegetables," she explained. "In 1995, it was found in human guts. The metabolic pathways in our kids are corrupt." [298]

Lalama says the increased exposure to Bt modified foods helps explain the jump in autism rates. "Bt also accounts for the disappearing bees, bats, and monarch butterflies. Surviving bees have been studied and found to have lost their ability to communicate with each other. Sounds just like our kids, yes?"

Her research has led her to a supplement called bitter orange which contains octopamine, a neurotransmitter found in the octopus and in bees. "We gave it to our kids. In 24 hours, we saw big changes in our children. A week later we got sentences." Lalama suggests that octopamine replaces communication abilities taken away by Bt-modified foods. [299]Whether you are concerned for yourself and family or even for your pet, shopping carefully and being aware of the food we eat is important. Look for the USDA Organic certification label on foods, as GM foods are not labeled as such at

---

[298] LaLama, A. (2009) Reversing Autism: Connecting the pieces with the latest research on Bt, Hg, Octopamine, Succinic acid, B12, Leptu and BIRM. Retrieved from: http://www.autismone.com/content/reversing-autism-connecting-pieces-latest-research-bthg-octopamine-succinic-acid-b12-leptu-
[299] LaLama, A. (2009) Reversing Autism: Connecting the pieces with the latest research on Bt, Hg, Octopamine, Succinic acid, B12, Leptu and BIRM. Retrieved from: http://www.autismone.com/content/reversing-autism-connecting-pieces-latest-research-bthg-octopamine-succinic-acid-b12-leptu-

this time. It is very difficult to determine what foods do not contain GM ingredients. Avoid foods that contain corn and soy products (including cooking oils), since these are most likely to have come from GE/GM crops.

# Chapter 8
# Feeding the Brain
# for Peak
# Performance

Fueling the body with clean food is imperative. The food you eat helps your body to build and rebuild itself continually at the cellular level. Individual cells live approximately 4 months; they then die and are replaced with new cells. As these new cells are created from the nutrients in your body, the old adage "you are what you eat" is quite literally true.

Your brain consumes roughly 20 percent of your daily calories. It demands a constant supply of glucose—primarily obtained from carbohydrates (fruits, vegetables, grains etc.). However, when muscles work hard, they also produce lactic acid, or lactate, as a byproduct. [300]

Researchers, in Denmark and The Netherlands, studied blood running to and from the heads of volunteers engaged in strenuous exercise. [301] The blood on its way

---

[300]Frankenfield, D., Roth-Yousey, L., & Compher. C. (May 2005) Comparison of Predictive Equations for Resting Metabolic Rate in Healthy Nonobese and Obese Adults: A Systematic Review. *American Journal of Clinical Nutrition 105*(5),775-789.

[301] Oikawa, K., Iizuka, K., Murakami, T., Nagai, T., Okita,K., Yonezawa, K., et al (2004) *Molecular and Cellular Biochemistry, 259,* (1-2), 151-156, DOI: 10.1023/B:MCBI.0000021366.62189.9d

to the brain was found to contain considerably more lactate than blood flowing from the brain. Further investigation showed that the brain was not *storing* the lactate from the muscles, but rather was using it as fuel. In fact, the brain helped to clear lactate from the circulation, thereby providing glucose to muscles that needed it for the hard work they were performing. [302]

These findings help explain why your brain is able to work properly when your body's demand for fuel and oxygen is at its highest. According to Leigh Gibson of Roehampton University in England, "The more recently evolved areas of the brain, such as the frontal cortex, are particularly sensitive to falling glucose levels, while brain areas regulating vital functions are hardier; when your glucose level drops, the symptom is confused thinking, not a change in breathing pattern." [303] This is not to suggest that consumption of large amounts of glucose is the answer. According to Marc Montminy of the Salk Institute for Biological Studies in California, "On the contrary, high glucose levels slowly but surely damage cells everywhere in the body, including those in the brain". [304]

In fact, the brain may even react to excess food as if it were a pathogen. According to Dongsheng Cai and his

---

[302] Klarlund PedersenB. &Hoffman-Goetz, L.Exercise and the Immune System: Regulation, Integration, and Adaptation *Physiol Rev July 1, 2000 80:1055-1081*

[303] Gibson, E. L. (2007) Carbohydrates and mental function: feeding or impeding the brain? Nutrition Bulletin, 32 Suppl., 71-83.

[304] Salk Institute For Biological Studies (2008) Food For Thought– Regulating Energy Supply To The Brain During Fasting. Press Release. Retrieved From Http://Www.Salk.Edu/News/Pressrelease_Details.Php?Press_Id=318

colleagues at the University of Wisconsin, the resulting immune response to excess food, (irrespective of weight gain) may cause cognitive deficits such as those associated with Alzheimer's disease.[305] Similarly, high blood sugar, coupled with a cognitive task, is associated with elevated cortisol — a hormone known to impair memory in high doses,

So what does all this mean to an athlete? It means the foods you consume must be high quality. In other words, food that gives the body maximum energy. Carbohydrates, fats and protein all work together to provide energy for the body. Complex carbohydrates are important in creating short term energy; fats create a more sustained long term energy source and proteins work more to build and rebuild.

To help you understand which foods are really high quality, foods can be assessed by what is called "nutrient density".[306] This is the amount of nutrition per calorie. The more nutrition in the fewer calories, the better the food is for you. For example, a Big Mac has some vitamins and minerals and protein and about 600 calories. However, two cups of spinach, one quarter cantaloupe and two eggs on whole grain bread have more nutrition, less than 300 calories and none of the unhealthy ingredients of the Big Mac (cholesterol,

---

[305] Zhang, X., Zhang, G., Zhang, H., Karin, M., Bai, H. & Cai, D. (2008, f-Kb    r Stress Link Overnutrition To Energy Imbalance And Obesity. Cell, 135 ( 1), 61-73, 3 October 2008.

[306] Darmon, N., Darmon, M., Maillot, M. & Drewnowski, A. (2005) A Nutrient Density Standard for Vegetables and Fruits: Nutrients per Calorie and Nutrients per Unit Cost. *Journal of the American Dietetic Association*.105 (12) 1881-1887.

saturated fats and total fat, toxic chemicals, hormones and antibiotics in the meat, corn syrup, etc.). [307]

For the athlete, increased activity for workouts, training or competition requires extra energy intake of these high quality foods. Dietary plans that provide the most efficient energy sources will help the athlete train and compete more efficiently. [308]The type, intensity and frequency of training as well as the size, age and sex of the individual are major factors that dictate energy needs. For example, "weekend" athletes who engage in short bursts of activity will have different energy needs than serious marathon runners who are intensely training.[309]

## CARBOHYDRATES

Sports nutritionists recommend about 55 to 65 percent of an athlete's calorie intake come from carbohydrates. Complex carbohydrates such as starches should make up the majority of carbohydrate fuel. Examples of starchy foods are breads, cereals, pastas, starchy vegetables such as corn and potatoes, and dried beans and peas. Fruits are also excellent sources of carbohydrates. It is important to eat a variety.[310], [311]

---

[307] Calorie Count (2013) http://caloriecount.about.com/calories-big-mac-i21111

[308] Anderson, J., L. Young & Prior, S.(2010) Nutrition for the Athlete. *Colorado State University Extension.* 9.362.

[309] Boeckner, L. (1998) Nutrition and the Athlete: Fueling Your Sport. *Nebraska Cooperative Extension* NF92-73.

[310] Shryer,D. (2007) *Peak Performance: Sports Nutrition.* Benchmark Books:Terrytown, NY.

[311] O'Neill, C. B. & Akintunde, P. G. (June 1, 2008) Optimizing Athletes' Performance Excellence and Wellness Through Nutrition and Exercise. Retrieved from: http://ssrn.com/abstract=1595403

Besides providing energy, carbohydrate-rich foods such as grain and cereal products, fruits, vegetables, and legumes are also an excellent source of fiber. Vitamins and minerals are abundant in many of these foods.[312]

In an athletic event, carbohydrates are used by the body as the initial fuel source. In short-burst, high-intensity events such as sprinting, jumping and pole vaulting, carbohydrates provide 100 percent of energy. For longer events fats are used along with the carbohydrates as the energy source.[313]

The body stores limited amounts of carbohydrates as glycogen. Through physical training and a diet rich in complex carbohydrates, athletes are able to store more glycogen and to use its limited supply sparingly. The amount of energy available from glycogen storage is about 1800 - 2000 calories. When the body runs low, athletes become fatigued and performance suffers.[314]

## Carbohydrate Loading

Carbohydrate loading (also called glycogen loading) is a technique that is commonly used by endurance athletes such as marathon runners, biathletes and

[312] CDC (2013) Carbohydrates. Retrieved from: http://www.cdc.gov/nutrition/everyone/basics/carbs.html

[313] Burke, L.M. (1997) Nutrition for post-exercise recovery. *Aust. J. Sci. Med. Sport* 29(1):3-10, March 1997.

[314] Shryer,D. (2007) *Peak Performance: Sports Nutrition.* Benchmark Books:Terrytown, NY.

triathletes.[315] It is important to note that this technique does not benefit athletes who are involved in training or competition for less than 90 continuous minutes. Fat in an endurance athlete's diet is kept to a minimum. It is recommended that an athlete receive no more than 30% of their calories from fat as its digestion and breakdown cannot supply energy fast enough. With this in mind, an endurance athlete should receive 60-70% of their calories from carbohydrates and the typical diet is therefore high in complex carbohydrates, moderate in protein and low in fat.[316]

The modified carbohydrate loading allows athletes to eat their normal high carbohydrate training diet. In the final three days prior to competition, athletes push daily carbohydrate intake to 525-550 grams of carbohydrate or 65 percent of calories from carbohydrate, whichever is greater. This final push of carbohydrate will enhance glycogen storage within the body. Intakes above 500 to 600 grams of carbohydrate per day do not contribute significantly to muscle glycogen storage or athletic performance.[317]

Some athletes prefer not to add carbohydrates to their diet. Instead they train less days before a competition

---

[315] Hawley, J.A. & Burke, L.M. Effect of meal frequency and timing on physical performance. *Br. J. Nutr.* 77 Suppl 1:S91-S103, April 1997.
[316] Burton, A. (2011). Nutrition for the Endurance Athlete: The Marathoners Diet for Optimal Performance. Marathon Guide.com. *Web Marketing Association 2010-2011* retrieved from http://www.marathonguide.com/training/articles/Nutrition.cfm
[317] Australian Sports Commission (2004) AIS Sports Nutrition Fact Sheet. Retrieved from http://www.triathlonandmultisportcoaching.com.au/docs/carbohydrateloading.pdf

thus using the extra 500-1,000 calories they would have burned during training to fuel their muscles.

## CARBOHYDRATES DURING AND AFTER ATHLETIC EVENTS

When athletic events last more than 60 minutes, athletes benefit by eating carbohydrates during exercise. The extra fuel helps them stay competitive longer. Slightly sweetened beverages which contain less than 24 grams of carbohydrate per one cup (8 oz) may be used. Nutritionists recommend 50-60 grams of carbohydrates per hour to fuel athletes through endurance events. Fruit juices that are diluted one part juice to one part water or some sports drinks will do the trick for endurance athletes.[318]

Following training or competition, nutritionists also recommend athletes eat complex carbohydrate-rich foods as soon as possible. After replenishment athletes can then resume their normal high carbohydrate training diet. Glycogen stores used for energy during activity also need to be replenished. [319]

## FATS

The other important fuel source for the athlete is fat. Compared to carbohydrates, fats have over twice as many calories as an equal weight of carbohydrate. During aerobic training, the body increases its ability to

---

[318] Driskell, J.A. & Wolinsky, I. (2009) Nutritional Concerns in Recreation, Exercise, and Sport. CRC Press:Boca Raton, FL.
[319] Shryer,D. (2007) *Peak Performance: Sports Nutrition*. Benchmark Books:Terrytown, NY.

use fat as an energy source so that glycogen can be spared. However, even in the best trained athletes, carbohydrates must always be available as a fuel source since fats cannot be used as the only fuel. [320]

Even though fats are an important fuel, it is not always necessary to add more fats to an existing diet as the body's fat storage is more than adequate to provide the extra energy. Even in a fairly lean individual, there will always be stored fat to provide a good energy source. For example, a 150-pound athlete who has 10 percent body fat has about 62,000 calories as stored energy. That's plenty of energy to fuel an athletic event over an extended period.[321] In fact, a diet that is moderately low in fat (no more than 30 percent of total calories from fat) will not hinder performance and will promote an eating style that will be beneficial throughout life.

## PROTEINS

When muscle glycogen is adequate, protein contributes only about 5% of the overall energy needed to maintain racing intensity.[322] Further, it is only burned as energy when glycogen depletion has occurred. Because protein is not able to supply as much energy as carbohydrates, it is considered an expensive and inefficient energy source.

---

[320] Burton, A. (2011). Nutrition for the Endurance Athlete: The Marathoners Diet for Optimal Performance. Marathon Guide.com. *Web Marketing Association 2010-2011* retrieved from http://www.marathonguide.com/training/articles/Nutrition.cfm
[321] Boeckner, L. (1998) Nutrition and the Athlete: Fueling Your Sport. *Nebraska Cooperative Extension* NF92-73.
[322] Gibala, M. (2007) Protein metabolism and endurance exercise. (conference paper). *Sports Medicine* 37(4) 337-341.

However, protein is predominantly responsible for muscle repair and maintenance. Whey protein's amino acid profile contains the highest percentage of essential amino acids (25%). These amino acids (leucine, isoleucine and valine) are most important for muscle repair.[323] Thus, consuming a good source of whey protein after a training session is critical in ensuring an athlete is able to recover quickly, and helps maintain their training frequency. Athletes that fail to consume adequate protein for recovery become susceptible to fatigue, anemia and lethargy.[324]

## FOOD AND THE BRAIN

Research on how food affects the brain and behavior is relatively new, however we now know that particular nutrients alter the brain chemistry causing changes in brain function, mood and behavior. The truth is what we eat has a direct effect on the production of chemical and their signals in the brain.[325] New technologies are being used to see this change with high tech neural imaging. Behavioral tests that measure motor and cognitive skills—or lack thereof—are also providing insights. Yet the science of nutrition and brain function is still evolving.

---

[323] Nutritional Supplement Review (2011) Whey Protein: Macronutrient. Retrieved from www.nutros.net/nrs-2015.html
[324] Burton, A. (2011). Nutrition for the Endurance Athlete: The Marathoners Diet for Optimal Performance. Marathon Guide.com. *Web Marketing Association 2010-2011* retrieved from http://www.marathonguide.com/training/articles/Nutrition.cfm
[325] Wolpert, S. & Wheeler, M. (2008) Food As Brain Medicine. *UCLA, UCLA Mag.* Jul 9, 2008.

## Boosting Neuronal Function

Chemical neurotransmitters such as norepinephrine, serotonin and dopamine allow the brain's billions of neurons to talk to one another through neural pathways. The ability to constantly replenish these neurons and connections is what keeps our brains healthy.[326]

However, as the brain ages, some function loss is seen as one starts to experience mild memory loss, lower cognition and slower brain speed. Some say the brain loses neurons faster than it can replace them and so loses function. However, neuroscientist James Joseph, neuroscientist from the Neuroscience Laboratory at the Jean Mayer USDA Human Nutrition Research Center on Aging (HNRCA) at Tufts University in Boston says, "Loss of mental agility may be less due to loss of brain cells than to the cells' failure to communicate effectively."[327] Joseph adds, "Vitamins and minerals in plant foods provide protective antioxidants. But fruits, vegetables, nuts, seeds, and grains contain thousands of other types of compounds that contribute significantly to the overall dietary intake of antioxidants. A partial measure of the antioxidant effect is called 'ORAC,' for Oxygen Radical Absorbance Capacity. ORAC scores are now showing up in charts and on some food and

---

[326] Markus, C.R., Olivier, B., Panhuysen, G., Gugten, J., van de Alles, M.,Westenberg, H., et al.( 2000)The bovine protein alpha-lactalbumin increases the plasma and in vulnerable subjects it raises brain serotonin activity, reduces cortisol and improves mood under stress. American Journal of Clinical Nutrition 71,1536–1544

[327] Joseph, J.A. (2007) Nutrition and Brain Function. Agricultural Research magazine.Aug 2007.

beverage packages. They may be helpful in choosing foods to include in your diet."[328] Antioxidants have been shown to be beneficial in neuronal protection and even reversal of neuronal connection loss.[329]

## B VITAMINS AND BRAIN POWER

All B vitamins are typically found grouped together in foods. Therefore, they're called B complex vitamins. Vitamin B complex includes seven vitamins: B1, B2, B3, B5, B6, B9 and B12. They're water-soluble and should be replenished every day with foods. [330]

An athlete needs B vitamins to help release energy from the foods they eat by converting proteins, carbohydrates and fats into fuel thereby increasing energy and strength. When there is a deficiency in these vital vitamins, the brain can experience brain fog, lack of coordination, depression and insomnia.

Sugar, caffeine, alcohol and nicotine as well as medications and stress can destroy B vitamins. A significant amount of B vitamins are also lost during the storing and cooking processes of foods because they're extremely sensitive to light and heat. Therefore

---

[328] Bliss, R.M. (Aug. 2011) Nutrition & brain function: food for the aging mind. *Agricultural Research*. Retrieved from: http://findarticles.com/p/articles/mi_m3741/is_7_55/ai_n27343330/
[329] Milgram NW, Head E, Muggenburg B, Holowachuk D, Murphey H, Estrada CJ, et al.(2002) Landmark discrimination learning in the dog: effects of age, an antioxidant fortified diet, and cognitive strategy. Neurosci Biobehav Rev 2002;26:679–95.
[330] Whitney, N; Rolfes, S Crowe, T Cameron-Smith, D Walsh, A (2011). *Understanding Nutrition*. Melbourne: Cengage Learning.

an athlete must protect the B vitamins in his system and foods to get the most benefit.[331]

The nervous system is also nourished by B vitamins, especially B1 and B12. When there is a deficiency of these vitamins, nervous system damage can occur causing increased irritability, numbness and weakness in hands and feet. [332]

Athletes, the elderly, vegatarians, pregnant and nursing women as well as those on birth control pills are most at risk for vitamin B deficiency. Alcoholics as well as those who eat an overabundance of sweets, refined and processed foods and very little fresh vegetables, fruits and whole grains, are also at risk for vitamin B deficiency. [333]

For athletes it is especially important to fill the diet with vitamin rich foods and, avoid those things that destroy B vitamins in your system.

## *VITAMIN B1*

Vitamin B1 (Thiamin) affects the nervous system and mental faculties. Thiamin is very important for the blood formation, carbohydrate metabolism and proper digestion. Also our bodies and minds need it for the energy, growth and learning capacity.

---

[331] Gropper, S; Smith, J (2009). *Advanced nutrition and human metabolism*. Belmont, CA: Cengage Learning.
[332] Fattal-Valevski, A (2011). "Thiamin (vitamin B1)". *Journal of Evidence-Based Complementary & Alternative Medicine* **16** (1): 12–20.
[333] NIH (2013) Vitamin B12. Office of Dietary Supplements. Retrieved from: http://ods.od.nih.gov/factsheets/VitaminB12-HealthProfessional/?print=1

Sources of thiamin in your diet are: meats, liver, fish, whole grains, beans and peas, nuts and seeds, yeast. The best vitamin B1 foods are: yeast, pork, green peas, soybean flour, sunflower seeds. [334]

## VITAMIN B2

Vitamin B2 (Riboflavin) is required for energy production. Freshness and vitality is exchanged for fatigue with lack of Vitamin B2. This vitamin is important in the metabolism of carbohydrates, fats and proteins. Also vitamin B2 is necessary for hemoglobin formation.

Riboflavin is present in all animal and plant origin products. The richest vitamin B2 foods are: beef and chicken liver and their hearts, meat, poultry, milk and yogurt. Other good sources of this B vitamin are: leafy green vegetables, avocado, egg yolks, cheese, beans and peas, whole grains. [335]

## VITAMIN B3

Vitamin B3 (Niacin) is involved in hormone synthesis. Another one of its function is creating energy from the foods. Emotional balance and body energy depend on this vitamin. Niacin involved in tissue breathing and that's why it is essential for healthy skin. It's very important for the nervous system and digestive system. Niacin lowers cholesterol and improves circulation.

---

[334] Combs, G. F. Jr. (2008) *The vitamins: Fundamental Aspects in Nutrition and Health*. 3rd Edition. Ithaca, NY: Elsevier Academic Press.
[335] Ball, G. (2006) Riboflavin in Vitamins in Foods, Analysis, Bioavailability, and Stability. Taylor and Francis Group, New York.

The best sources of vitamin B3 in your diet are: liver, chicken breast, yeast, rice and wheat germs, fresh green peas, and avocado. Meat, fish, milk, fresh vegetables and fruits, mushrooms, grains and grain products, peas and beans.[336]

## VITAMIN B5

Vitamin B5 (Pantothenic acid) is required by all sells that make up our body. Known as "the anti-stress vitamin", it helps to convert fats, carbohydrates, and proteins into energy. Vitamin B5 is involved in metabolic functions and its deficiency may lead to an increase in body weight. Also, it supports the work of the heart and improves the brain function. Vitamin B5 considered as the one of the best nutrients for slimming and against aging.

The richest food sources of pantothenic acid are: liver, yeast, meats, wheat germ, sunflower seeds and peanuts.

Whole grains are another good source of the vitamin, but milling often removes much of B5 vitamin, as it is found in the outer layers of whole grains. Broccoli and avocados and other green leafed vegetables also have an abundance of panthothenic acid. [337]

---

[336] Zellner, C., Pullinger, C.R., Aouizerat, B.E., *et al.* (2005) Variations in human HM74 (GPR109B) and HM74A (GPR109A) niacin receptors. *Hum. Mutat.* **25** (1): 18–21. doi:10.1002/humu.20121
[337] MedlinePlus (2007) *Pantothenic acid (Vitamin-B5), Dexpanthenol.* Natural Standard Research Collaboration. U.S. National Library of Medicine.

## VITAMIN B6

Vitamin B6 (Pyridoxine) affects both physical and mental health. This is anti-depressant vitamin because it helps to synthesize substances that are responsible for the appetite, good mood, and good sleep. It is necessary for the absorption of fats and protein. It promotes the formation of red blood cells and vitamin B6 is required by the nervous system and brain for normal brain function.

All foods contain some vitamin B6.The best vitamin B6 sources are: beef liver, chicken breast and liver, avocado, banana, unpeeled potato, meats and yeast. Other sources include eggs, fish, spinach, peas, broccoli, carrots, sunflower seeds, walnuts, wheat germ, whole grains. [338]

## VITAMIN B9

Vitamin B9 (Folic acid, Folate) plays a very important role in growth and formation of the human body. Therefore, it is essential during pregnancy. Folic acid involved not only in the fetal development, but in the mother's recovery also. It is needed for energy production and the formation of red blood cells. Deficiency of this vitamin can lead to anemia. [339]

---

[338] Combs, G.F. (2008) The Vitamins: Fundamental Aspects in Nutrition and Health. San Diego: Elsevier.

[339] Smith AD, Kim YI, Refsum H. Is folic acid good for everyone? *Am J Clin Nutr.* 2008;87(3):517-33.

## Sources

Folic acid present in great amounts in leafed vegetables, nuts and seeds, meat, fish, and eggs. The richest vitamin B9 foods are: chicken liver, beef liver, avocado, beans and peas, sunflower seeds, yeast. [340]

## VITAMIN B12

Vitamin B12 differs from other B vitamins in the way that it cannot be found in plants, but present in animal origin products only. Our body requires a very small amount of this vitamin. Symptoms indicating the deficiency of vitamin B12 show up five or six years later. [305]

This vitamin is needed to prevent anemia, because it plays an important role in formation of red blood cells and in utilization of iron. Also vitamin B12 prevents nerve damage, required for proper digestion, absorption of foods, and aids in the metabolism of carbohydrates and fats. [341]

Vitamin B12 is found in foods that come from animals, including fish and shellfish, meat (especially liver), poultry, eggs, milk, and milk products. Chicken liver,

---

[340] National Academy of Sciences. Institute of Medicine. Food and Nutrition Board., ed (1998). "Chapter 4 - Thiamin". *Dietary Reference Intakes for Thiamin, Riboflavin, Niacin, Vitamin B₆, Folate, Vitamin B₁₂, Pantothenic Acid, Biotin, and Choline*. Washington, D.C.: National Academy Press. 58–86.
[341] National Academy of Sciences. Institute of Medicine. Food and Nutrition Board., ed (1998). "Chapter 4 - Thiamin". *Dietary Reference Intakes for Thiamin, Riboflavin, Niacin, Vitamin B₆, Folate, Vitamin B₁₂, Pantothenic Acid, Biotin, and Choline*. Washington, D.C.: National Academy Press. 58–86.

beef liver and clams are the richest sources of vitamin B12. [342]

Although we need this vitamin in small amounts, it is important as the air we breathe. If your diet excludes animal products, than you need to replenish vitamin B12 with supplements.[343]

A recent study by epidemiologists Paul Jacques and Martha Morris, biochemist Jacob Selhub, and physician Irwin H. Rosenberg, who heads the Nutrition and Neurocognition Laboratory at the Jean Mayer USDA Human Nutrition Research Center on Aging (HNRCA) at Tufts University in Boston, Massachusetts, showed the interrelationships among the B vitamins (known to be involved in the synthesis of chemicals crucial to brain function) and cognitive function in this age of folate fortification. Scientists have long known that being seriously deficient in vitamin B12 leads to impaired cognitive function due to neurological complications. The researchers used a combination of blood markers to classify subjects' vitamin B12 ranking.[344]

---

[342] Paoloni-Giacobino, A., Grimble, R. & Pichard, C. (2003) Genetics and nutrition. *Clinical Nutrition.* Vol 22, Issue 5, Pages 429-435 (October 2003)

[343] NIH (2013) Vitamin B12. Office of Dietary Supplements. Retrieved from: http://ods.od.nih.gov/factsheets/VitaminB12-HealthProfessional/?print=1

[344] M.S. Morris; P.F. Jacques; I.H. Rosenberg; J. Selhub (2010) Circulating unmetabolized folic acid and 5-methyltetrahydrofolate in relation to anemia, macrocytosis, and cognitive test performance in American seniors. *American Journal of Clinical Nutrition* (2010) 91, (1733-44))                    2010;92(4):1002-.

Morris, who led the study, found that among people aged 60 and older, those with high blood levels of folate and normal, or adequate, vitamin B12 status scored high on cognitive function tests. These seniors were given a test that required response speed, in addition to attentiveness, visual-spatial skills, associative learning, and memory.

But what about those who had low vitamin B12 blood levels—a status that is common among seniors due to the poorer gastrointestinal conditions that come with aging? Low vitamin B12 status was linked with lower scores on cognitive tests.

"The people with high folate and low B12 status were more likely to exhibit both cognitive impairment and anemia than those with normal folate and low B12 status," says Jacques.[345]

## LOSS OF B VITAMINS IN FOODS

We know most B vitamins are very sensitive to light and heat and can be destroyed easily during cooking, freezing and storage.

If you think you're not getting enough B vitamins in your diet alone, vitamin B supplements might be the answer. If supplements are called for, remember the B vitamins work together so should always be taken together. If you are deficient in one, most likely you are deficient in another.

---

[345] USDA (2007) Boosting Our Knowledge of Brain Food. *Agricultural Research*. In: *Human Nutrition,*
an ARS national program (#107)retrieved from:www.nps.ars.usda.gov.

## VITAMIN D

Vitamin D is a fat-soluble vitamin that is naturally present in very few foods; therefore it is most commonly added to other foods or taken as a dietary supplement.[346] While it is well recognized that vitamin D is necessary for optimal bone health, emerging evidence is finding that adequate vitamin D intake reduces risk for conditions such as stress fracture, total body inflammation, infectious illness, and impaired muscle function.[347] Studies in athletes have found that vitamin D status is variable and is dependent on outdoor training time (during peak sunlight), skin color, and geographic location. Although research has found that athletes generally do not meet the U.S. dietary reference intake for vitamin D.[348]

Foods that do provide some amounts of Vitamin D are; the flesh of fatty fish (such as salmon, tuna, and mackerel) and fish liver oils are among the best sources.[349],[350] Small amounts of vitamin D are found in

---

[346] Holick, M.F. (March 2006). "High prevalence of vitamin D inadequacy and implications for health". *Mayo Clin. Proc.* 81 (3): 353–73. doi:10.4065/81.3.353

[347] Pittas, A.G., Chung, M., Trikalinos, T., Mitri, J., Brendel, M., Patel, K. et al (Mar 2010). "Vitamin D and Cardiometabolic Outcomes: A Systematic Review". *Annals of internal medicine* 152 (5): 307–14. doi:10.1059/0003-4819-152-5-201003020-00009

[348] Larson-Meyer, D.E. & Willis, K.S. ( 2010 Jul-Aug) Vitamin D and athletes. CURR SPORTS MED REP.;9(4):220-6. REVIEW. PMID:20622540

[349] Institute of Medicine, Food and Nutrition Board. (2010) Dietary Reference Intakes for Calcium and Vitamin D. Washington, DC: National Academy Press.

[350] U.S. Department of Agriculture, Agricultural Research Service. (2010) Retrieved from: USDA National Nutrient Database for Standard Reference, Release 23.

beef liver, cheese, and egg yolks. Vitamin D in these foods is primarily in the form of vitamin D3 and its metabolite 25(OH) D$_3$.[351] Some mushrooms provide vitamin D$_2$ in variable amounts. [352],[353] Mushrooms with enhanced levels of vitamin D$_2$ from being exposed to ultraviolet light under controlled conditions are also available.

Fortified foods provide most of the vitamin D in the American diet. [354],[355] For example, almost all of the U.S. milk supply is voluntarily fortified with 100 IU/cup. [356] In the 1930s, a milk fortification program was implemented in the United States to combat rickets, then a major public health problem. Other dairy products made from milk, such as cheese and ice cream, are generally not fortified. Ready-to-eat breakfast cereals often contain added vitamin D, as do

[351] Ovesen L, Brot C, Jakobsen J. Food contents and biological activity of 25-hydroxyvitamin D: a vitamin D metabolite to be reckoned with? Ann Nutr Metab 2003;47:107-13

[352] Mattila PH, Piironen VI, Uusi-Rauva EJ, Koivistoinen PE. Vitamin D contents in edible mushrooms. J Agric Food Chem 1994;42:2449-53.

[353] Calvo MS, Whiting SJ, Barton CN. Vitamin D fortification in the United States and Canada: current status and data needs. Am J Clin Nutr 2004;80:1710S-6S.

[354] Institute of Medicine, Food and Nutrition Board. (2010)Dietary Reference Intakes for Calcium and Vitamin D. Washington, DC: National Academy Press,

[355] Calvo MS, Whiting SJ, Barton CN. Vitamin D fortification in the United States and Canada: current status and data needs. Am J Clin Nutr 2004;80:1710S-6S.

[356] Holick, M.F., Binkley, N.C., Bischoff-Ferrari, H.A., Gordon, C.M., Hanley, D.A., Heaney, R.P. et al (2011) Evaluation, treatment, and prevention of vitamin D deficiency: an Endocrine Society clinical practice guideline. *J Clin Endocrinol Metab* 96 (7): 1911–30. doi:10.1210/jc.2011-0385

some brands of orange juice, yogurt, margarine and other food products.[357]

## *VITAMIN E*

Vitamin E is a fat-soluble vitamin found in many foods, fats, and oils and is an antioxidant. This vitamin is important in the formation of red blood cells and helps the body to use vitamin K.[358]

In 2004 at the Linus Pauling Institute at Oregon State University, researchers found that ultra-marathon runners who used supplements of vitamins E for six weeks prior to their races, prevented the increase in lipid oxidation that is otherwise associated with extreme exercise. Although the type of metabolic damage observed in these runners is often found after heart attacks, strokes, surgery and other traumas, the researchers noted that this study provides more evidence that supplementation of vitamin E as an antioxidant, can help prevent damaging lipid oxidation and other health concerns associated with it.[359]

In 2010, Dr. Ali Razmkon, a neurosurgery resident at the Shiraz (Iran) University of Medical Sciences, found high doses of Vitamin E given after a traumatic brain

---

[357] Lerch, C., Meissne, T.& Lerch, C. (2007) Interventions for the prevention of nutritional rickets in term born children. In Lerch, Christian. *Cochrane database of systematic reviews (Online)* (4): CD006164. doi:10.1002/14651858.CD006164.pub2
[358] Brigelius-Flohe, B & Traber (1999) Vitamin E: function and metabolism. *FASEB* 13: 1145–1155.
[359] Oregon State University (2004, July 15). Study Shows Vitamins C And E Can Prevent Metabolic Damaage In Extreme Exercise. ScienceDaily. Retrieved July 2, 2013, from http://www.sciencedaily.com /releases/2004/07/040715080010.htm

injury cut in-hospital mortality rates 29% as opposed to those patients receiving either high or low doses of Vitamin C or a placebo.[360] For his work on the trial, Dr. Razmkon won the Synthes Resident Award for Research on Brain and Craniofacial Injury.

## SUPPLEMENTS FOR CONCUSSION AND TBIS

Athletes are prime candidates for head injury. Even though most athletes don't consider mild head trauma an issue, more and more information is coming out about cumulative effects of even mild head injuries over time. There are vitamins and supplements that can actually help the brain heal faster and minimize long-term issues.[361]

Free radicals are formed at some point in almost every mechanism of secondary brain injury. These highly reactive molecules attack the fatty acids in the myelin and cell-membrane. If left unchecked, lipid peroxidation, an indicator of oxidative stress in tissues and cells, spreads over the surface of the cell membrane and eventually leads to cell death. [362]Antioxidants are therefore important to

---

[360] Razmkon, A., Sadidi, A., Sherafat-Kazemzadeh, E., Mehrafshan, A &, Bakhtazad, A. (2010) Beneficial Effects of Vitamin C and Vitamin E Administration in Severe Head Injury: A Randomized Double-Blind Controlled Trial: 931. *Neurosurgery,67* (2) 546. doi: 10.1227/01.NEU.0000387003.89378.

[361] Brain Injury Association of America (2007) *The Essential Brain Injury Guide* (4th ed). Ypsilanti, MI: Rainbow Rehabilitation Centers, Inc.

[362] O'Connell, K.M. & Littleton-Kearney, M.T. (2013) The Role of Free Radicals in Traumatic Brain Injury. *Biol Res Nurs.* 2013 Jul;15(3):253-63. doi: 10.1177/1099800411431823.

recovery as well as prevention in protecting the brain after an injury. [363]

There are several vitamin and supplement protocols given to those who have sustained head injuries. Intravenous Glutathione which is an important nutrient and energy source for the brain and acts as a major antioxidant within each cell can be helpful to heal brain injury.[364] Supplements rich in antioxidants (beta carotene, vitamin C, vitamin E, and selenium) can be utilized, to pump more oxygen to the brain and to hasten the healing process while at the same time preventing further deterioration internally after a concussion has been suffered. Vitamin C bolsters immune system function, and can decrease blood pressure, while preventing internal blood clots and bruising, thus greatly speeding recovery. Vitamin E is also beneficial for tissue repair. Therefore, these two vitamins, C and E, are more effective when used together. [365]

Meyer's cocktail which includes a combination of magnesium, calcium, vitamin B12, vitamin B6, Vitamin B5, Vitamin B Complex and Vitamin C can also be helpful.[366]

363 Jacobsson,S., Cassel, G.E. & Persson, S. (1999) Increased levels of nitrogen oxides and lipid peroxidation in the rat brain after soman-induced seizures. *Archives of Toxicology ,73*, 269-273, DOI: 10.1007/s002040050616

[364] Kidd, P.M. (1997) Glutathione: systemic protectant against oxidative and free radical damage. *Altern Med Rev*;2:155-176.

[365] Hall, E.D., Vaishnav, R.A. & Mustafa, A.G. (2010) Antioxident Therapies for Traumatic Brain Injury. *Neurotherapeutics.* 2010 Jan;7(1):51-61. doi: 10.1016/j.nurt.2009.10.021.

[366] Gaby, A. (2002) Intravenous nutrient therapy: the "Myers' cocktail". *Altern Med Rev* **7** (5): 389–403.

The B vitamins are necessary to maintain proper nerve function and help relieve symptoms such as depression and anxiety can accompany concussion. The B complex vitamin has the optimal effect, as all necessary B vitamins are present. Cellular damage caused by free radicals is prevented by the mineral selenium. Zinc, an antioxidant which is also an essential mineral for body function, helps keep the levels of vitamin E in the body at an optimum. Natural supplements can be used in addition to antioxidants or as supplements in their own right, these various natural supplements can reduce memory loss and its effects if used regularly. The coenzyme Q10 is also useful in transporting oxygen to the cells. [367]

Vitamins are not the only things helpful for TBI. Hyperbaric Oxygen Therapy treatments are also helpful in forcing more oxygen into the body under pressure and to dissolve in all the body's fluids. These fluids carry the extra oxygen to the damaged cells in the brain and help the healing process.[368]

Whether you need assistance with cognitive issues, you are a professional athletes or just trying to be fit, always shop carefully and be aware of the food you eat. The following table contains a list of nutrients, the foods they can be found in and how they affect cognition and emotion.

---

[367] Silver, J.M., MacAllister, T.W. & Yudofsky, S.C. (2011) *The Textbook of Traumatic Brain Injury*. American Psychiatric Pub: Arlington, VA.
[368] McDonagh, M., Helfand, M., Carson, S. & Russman, B.S. (2004) Hyperbaric oxygen therapy for traumatic brain injury: a systematic review of the evidence. *Arch Phys Med Rehabil* **85** (7): 1198–204.

| Nutrient | Effects on cognition and emotion | Food sources |
|---|---|---|
| **Omega-3 fatty acids** (for example, alpha-linolenic acid (ALA), eicosapentae noic acid (EPA), and docosahexae noic acid (DHA) | Reduces inflammation and help prevent risk factors associated with chronic diseases such as heart disease, cancer, and arthritis. These essential fatty acids are highly concentrated in the brain and appear to be particularly important for cognitive (brain memory and performance), to reduce depression,mood disorders, ADHD and behavioral function. | Fish, such as salmon, tuna, and halibut, other marine life such as algae and krill, certain plants (including purslane), and nut oils. |
| **Curcumin** | Amelioration of cognitive decay in mouse model of Alzheimer's disease; amelioration of cognitive decay in traumatic brain injury in rodents | Turmeric (curry spice) |
| **Flavonoids** | Cognitive enhancement in combination with exercise in rodents; improvement of cognitive function in the elderly | Cocoa, green tea, Ginkgo tree, citrus fruits, wine (higher in red wine), dark chocolate |
| **Saturated fat** | Promotion of cognitive decline in adult rodents; aggravation of cognitive impairment after brain trauma in rodents; exacerbation of cognitive decline in aging humans | Butter, ghee, suet, lard, coconut oil, cottonseed oil, palm kernel oil, |

| Nutrient | Effects on cognition and emotion | Food sources |
|---|---|---|
| | | dairy products (cream, cheese), meat |
| B vitamins | Supplementation with vitamin B6, vitamin B12 or folate has positive effects on memory performance in women of various ages; vitamin B12 improves cognitive impairment in rats fed a choline-deficient diet | Various natural sources. Vitamin B12 is not available from plant products |
| Vitamin D | Important for preserving cognition in the elderly | Fish liver, fatty fish, mushrooms, fortified products, milk, soy milk, cereal grains |
| Vitamin E | Amelioration of cognitive impairment after brain trauma in rodents, reduces cognitive decay in the elderly | Asparagus, avocado, nuts, peanuts, olives, red palm oil, seeds, spinach, vegetable oils, wheatgerm |
| Choline | Reduction of seizure-induced memory impairment in rodents; a review of the literature reveals | Egg yolks, soy beef, chicken, |

| Nutrient | Effects on cognition and emotion | Food sources |
|---|---|---|
| | evidence for a causal relationship between dietary choline and cognition in humans and rats | veal, turkey liver, lettuce |
| **Combination of vitamins (C, E, carotene)** | Antioxidant vitamin intake delays cognitive decline in the elderly | Vitamin C: citrus fruits, several plants and vegetables, calf and beef liver. Vitamin E: see above |
| **Calcium, zinc, selenium** | High serum calcium is associated with faster cognitive decline in the elderly; reduction of zinc in diet helps to reduce cognitive decay in the elderly; lifelong low selenium level associated with lower cognitive function in humans | Calcium: milk, coral. Zinc: oysters, a small amount in beans, nuts, almonds, whole grains, sunflower seeds. Selenium: nuts, cereals, meat, fish, eggs |

| Nutrient | Effects on cognition and emotion | Food sources |
|---|---|---|
| Copper | Cognitive decline in patients with Alzheimer's disease correlates with low plasma concentrations of copper | Oysters, beef/lamb liver, Brazil nuts, blackstrap molasses, cocoa, black pepper |
| Iron | Normalizes cognitive function in young women | Red meat, fish, poultry, lentils, beans |

## OMEGA-3 FATTY ACIDS

According to Gómez-Pinilla, a member of UCLA's Brain Research Institute and Brain Injury Research Center, omega-3 fatty acids, found in salmon, walnuts and kiwi fruit, provide many benefits. These benefits include improving learning and memory and helping to fight against such mental disorders as depression and mood disorders, schizophrenia, and dementia. Synapses in the brain connect neurons and provide critical functions such as learning and memory and are essential for brain function. If the body is deficient in Omege-3 fatty acids, there is an increased risk for several mental disorders including attention-deficit disorder, dyslexia, dementia, depression, bipolar disorder and schizophrenia.[369]

Children who had increased amounts of omega-3 fatty acids performed better in school, in reading and in spelling and had fewer behavioral problems. Preliminary studies done in England, show that school performance improved among a group of students receiving omega-3 fatty acids. In an Australian study, 396 children between the ages six and 12 who were given a drink with omega-3 fatty acids and other nutrients (iron, zinc, folic acid and vitamins A, B6, B12 and C) showed higher scores on tests measuring verbal intelligence and learning and memory after six months and one year than a control group of students who did not receive the nutritional drink. This study was also conducted with 394 children in Indonesia. The results showed higher test scores for boys and girls in Australia, but only for girls in Indonesia.[370]

One omega-3 fatty acid seems to be especially good for the brain. Docosahexaenoic acid, or DHA, is the most abundant omega-3 fatty acid in brain's cell membranes. It can be found in salmon and reduces oxidative stress and enhances synaptic plasticity and learning and memory. A healthy diet and exercise can reduce the effect of brain injury and lead to a better recovery. However, the brain and body are unable to make DHA;

[369] Gómez-Pinilla, F. (2008) Brain foods: the effects of nutrients on brain function. *Nature ReviewsNeuroscience 9,*568-578. doi:10.1038/nrn2421
[370] Wolpert, S., Wheeler, M. (2008) Food as brain medicine. *UCLA Magazine Online.* Retrieved http://magazine.ucla.edu

it has to come through our diet. Therefore a balanced diet rich in omega-3 fatty acids is essential.

Health is also genetic. Not only a healthy long life, but mental health can also be affected by the diet of the previous generations. A long-term study based on more than 100 years of birth, death, health and genealogical records for 300 Swedish families in an isolated village showed an individual's risk for diabetes and early death increased if his or her paternal grandparents grew up in times of food abundance rather than food shortage.[371]

Emerging research indicates that the effects of diet on the brain, combined with the effects of exercise and a good night's sleep, can strengthen synapses and provide other cognitive benefits.

## CONCLUSION

We are connected: Our bodies, our brains and what we use to fuel both. In today's world it is an ongoing struggle to keep out contaminants that are in our food and environment while still feeding the brain with adequate food to function.

Your brain cells need twice the energy of the other cells in your body. Neurons demand a high level of energy, as they all always in a state of metabolic activity. Even during sleep, neurons are still at work repairing and rebuilding their worn-out structural components. They

---

[371] University of California - Los Angeles (2008, July 11) Scientists Learn How Food Affects The Brain: Omega 3 Especially Important. *Science Daily*. Retrieved July 9, 2013, from http://www.sciencedaily.com /releases/2008/07/080709161922.htm

are also manufacturing enzymes and neurotransmitters that must be transported out to the very ends of their nerve branches, some that can be several inches, or even feet, away.[372]

Most demanding of a neuron's energy, however, are the bioelectric signals responsible for communication throughout the nervous system. This nerve transmission consumes one-half of all the brain's energy (nearly 10% of the whole body's energy). With this in mind, it's not hard to imagine that if we are feeding our body food that is toxic and devoid of nutrition how easily that translates to our brain function.[373]

[372] Brown, J. (2011) R3 Diet: Reverse, Retrain, Rebuild Your Body and Mind. Xlibris Corporation.

[373] Allen, C. (2009) Water and the Brain. Retrieved from: http://www.isisboston.com/assets/PDF-Files/Ionized-Water-and-the-Brain.pdf

# Chapter 9
# Neurofeedback
# History

Biofeedback is the basis for many of the neurotherapies we use today. Its subcategory, neurofeedback, is a based upon the same principles but looks at direct brain responses rather than on more remote biological signals. In this chapter we look back at biofeedback, the types of neurofeedback and their history.

## Biofeedback

According to the Association for Applied Psychophysiology and Biofeedback (AAPB), biofeedback is:

*A process that enables an individual to learn how to change physiological activity for the purposes of improving health and performance. Precise instruments measure physiological activity such as brainwaves, heart function, breathing, muscle activity, and skin temperature. These instruments rapidly and accurately 'feedback' information to the user. The presentation of this information—often in conjunction with changes in thinking, emotions, and behavior— supports desired physiological changes. Over time, these changes can endure without continued use of an instrument"*[374]

Biofeedback is a non-invasive, drug-free process that lets us receive real-time information about bodily functions such as heart rate, blood pressure and muscle tension. We use this physiological information to learn how to use our minds to gain control of physical processes previously considered an automatic response of the autonomous nervous system.

Biofeedback is actually an extension of the processes we use every day to manage our interactions with our environment. For example, when we touch a hot stove, the heat and pain sensors in our fingers register the sensation, feed it back to our brains and our brain directs our muscles to respond appropriately: we remove our hand from the hot surface. Moreover, we accomplish this without the need for conscious thought. We do not need to form the thought, "The stove is hot!" followed by a conscious direction to our arm and hand muscles, "Move your finger away from the stove!" It all happens subconsciously (and it's a good thing it does, too!). Just as our brains can automatically manage such environmental interactions that could threaten the integrity of our bodies, so too can our brains manage much more subtle body-environment interactions without the involvement of our conscious minds. With appropriate signals, our brains can control a wide variety of otherwise autonomous bodily functions. Yogic gurus have long shown their abilities to control their physiological

---

[374] Association for Applied Psychophysiology & Biofeedback (2008) What is biofeedback? Retrieved from: http://www.aapb.org/.

processes through meditation. You need not rise to this level, however, to gain some conscious control over your bodies' and brains' processes.

In Germany in the early 1900s, J. H. Schultz developed a technique called Autogenic Training,[375] in which verbal instructions were used to guide a person to a more relaxed and controlled, physiological state. By the 1930s, Edmund Jacobson in the United States developed a technique called Progressive Relaxation.[376] This was used to teach the difference between tension and relaxation by using a series of muscle activities. With this knowledge a person could effectively reduce tension and reduce the symptoms of stress related maladies.

The term Biofeedback, a word coined in the 1960s, was actually discovered in the 1940s as scientists were researching operant and classical conditioning for behavior modification (Jonas, 1973). They found their research subjects could be trained to alter brain activity, blood pressure, muscle tension, heart rate and other bodily functions that are not normally controlled voluntarily.[377]

By the 1960s, Neal Miller, Ph.D., of Rockefeller University, discovered that laboratory animals could be

---

[375] Stetter, F., Kupper, S. (March 2002) Autogenic training: a meta-analysis of clinical outcome studies. *Applied Psychophysiology and Biofeedback 27*(1), 45–98.
[376] Jacobson, E. (1938) *Progressive relaxation*. Chicago: University of Chicago Press.
[377] Lazarus, R. S. (1998) Fifty Years of the Research and Theory of R.S. Lazarus: An Analysis of Historical and Perennial Issues. Mahwah, New Jersey: Lawrence Erlbaum Associates.

trained to increase or decrease their heart rates by simply being rewarded for producing the desired physiological responses.[378] Later, by teaching six laboratory animals to blush only in the right ear and another six to blush only in the left, Miller was able to demonstrate that animals could learn to dilate specific blood vessels despite the fact that these organs are controlled by sympathetic (involuntary) nerves.

At the same time, other scientists worked with human subjects. Given feedback about specific automatic physiological responses of which they were normally unaware, these subjects were taught to modify or control functions such as heart rate and hand temperature.[379] Within the last 25 years, continued research has shown biofeedback to be a viable therapeutic tool in the treatment of many disorders, including headache, high blood pressure, muscle spasm, chronic anxiety, neuro-muscular dysfunction, epilepsy, insomnia, asthma and numerous other conditions.

## EEG NEUROFEEDBACK

Neurofeedback is biofeedback which is confined to brain function. [380] Electroencephalogram, or EEG, dates

---

[378] Jonas, Gerald. (1973) *Visceral Leaning.* New York: Viking Press.
[379] Yucha, C; Montgomery D (2008) *Evidence-based practice in biofeedback and neurofeedback.* Wheat Ridge, CO: AAPB.Retrieved from:
http://www.isnr.org/uploads/EvidenceBasedYuchaMontgomeryW.pdf.
[380] Masterpasqual, F. & Healey, K. N. ( 2003) Neurofeedback in psychological practice. *Professional Psychology: Research & Practice. 34* (6),652-656.

back to the mid to late nineteenth century.[381] In 1875, Richard Caton demonstrated his technique for detecting the electrical activity from the exposed surfaces of the brains of living rabbits and monkeys to a meeting of the British Medical Association and later published them in the British Medical Journal.[382] He is credited with the discovery of the spontaneous EEG in animals as well as demonstrating the ability to detect electrical brain responses to stimuli.

In 1924, Hans Berger, German psychiatrist, found small amounts of electrical current could be measured with electrodes connected to a person's scalp. He coined the term electroencephalogram as well.[383]

Further investigation proved that EEG could be used for biofeedback of brain activity and, in 1929; the first paper on the subject was published.[384] Early researchers focused on operant conditioning of alpha brain waves primarily for deep relaxation and meditation.[164] Operant conditioning refers to the use of consequences or reinforcement to change voluntary behavior. Our penal system is the primary institutional version of this concept.

In the 1960s, Barry Sterman of UCLA discovered that cats that had been trained with EEG biofeedback using

---

[381] Evans, J. R., & Abarbanel, A (1999) *Introduction to Quantitative EEG and Neurofeedback.*London: Academic Press.
[382] Finger, Stanley (2001) Origins of Neuroscience: A History of Explorations into Brain Function . USA: Oxford University Press.
[383] Schulte, B.P.M. (1970) *"Berger, Hans", Dictionary of Scientific Biography* .New York: Charles Scribner's Sons.
[384] Empson, J. (1986) Human Brainwaves:T he Psycological Significance of the Electroencephalogram. London: The Macmillan Press Ltd.

SMR/beta protocols (the middle to high frequency range, 12-20 Hz) from a previous unrelated experiment were immune from seizures when exposed to toxic chemicals that induced epileptic seizures and death in untreated cats.

This technique with EEG biofeedback using SMR/beta protocols on humans was replicated in more than twenty studies.[385] EEG neurofeedback is a type of operant conditioning in which an individual modifies the amplitude, frequency or coherence of his brain's electrical activity. The goal of EEG neurofeedback is to train the individual to normalize abnormal EEG frequencies. With this neurofeedback approach, the brain frequencies that are in excess are reduced, and those with a deficit are increased.[386]

The Site-Frequency Specificity and the Self-Regulating Brain models of neurofeedback training improve the ability of an individual to maintain homeostasis (or internal equilibrium) and to improve stability when responding to a sudden challenge or insult to the regulatory system.[387]

In the last 30 years, ongoing research using EEG neurofeedback has continued to show positive results

[385] Sterman, M. B. (2000) Basic concepts and clinical findings in the treatment of seizure disorders with EEG operant conditioning. *Clin Electroencephalogr* 31 :1: 45–55. PMID 10638352
[386] Hardt, J. V. (1975) The ups and downs of learning alpha feedback. *Proceedings, Biofeedback Research Society, 6*, Monterey.
[387] Othmer, S., Othmer, S. F., & Kaiser, D. A. (1999) EEG biofeedback: Training for ADHD and related disruptive behavior disorders. In J. A. Incorvaia & B. F. Mark-Goldstein, & D. Tessmer (Eds)., *Understanding, Diagnosing, & Treating ADHD in Children and Adolescents*. New York: Aronson.

in many areas including mood disorders, epilepsy, traumatic brain injury, sleep disorders, attention deficit disorders, autism and Post Traumatic Stress Disorder.[388],[389]

## HEG NEUROFEEDBACK

Remember that arteries bring oxygenated, glucose-rich blood from the lungs and heart and veins carry the "used" blood back to be replenished with oxygen and glucose in order to continuously fuel the body's activities. In the cells, including in the neurons that comprise the brain, glucose is converted to energy using oxygen.[390]

When a portion of the brain is activated, the demand for nutrients increases and more oxygen and glucose are called in to the specific area to help fuel the increased cellular activity.[391] Brain activity can also

---

[388] Hammond, D. C. (2005) Temporal lobes and their importance in neurofeedback. *Journal of Neurotherapy, 9* (1), 67-87. doi:10.1300/J184v09n01_08

[389] Levesque, J., Beauregard, M., & Mensour, B. (2006) Effect of neurofeedback training on the neural substrates of selective attention in children with attention- deficit/hyperactivity disorder: A functional magnetic resonance imaging study. *Neuroscience Letters, 394*(3), 216-221. doi:10.1300/J184v09n04_09

[390] Brooks, G. A., et al. (2005) *Exercise Physiology: Human Bioenergetics and Its Applications,4th ed.* New York: McGraw-Hill.

[391] Toomim, H., Mize, W., Kwong, P. C., & Toomim, M. (2004) Intentional increase of cerebral blood oxygenation using hemoencephalography (HEG). *Journal of Neurotherapy, 8* (3), 5-21. Retrieved from: http://www.biocompresearch.org/Tinius%20HEG%204%2012%2004.ht m

---

produce increased temperatures in the venous blood, as oxygenation of glucose produces heat.[392]

We often hear that we only use a small percentage of our brain. In truth, it's all used, just not all at the same time. If we used the entire brain at one time it would overheat and be severely damaged. The flow of blood cools the brain and prevents overheating.[393] Hemoencephalography neurofeedback is separate from and different than EEG neurofeedback. Rather than monitoring the brain's minute and complex electrical signals, as done in EEG neurofeedback, HEG monitors changing brain activity using either the local brain temperature or flow of oxygenated blood. This method is increasing in popularity among professionals struggling with the difficulties, noise issues and complex treatment protocols inherent in EEG neurofeedback.[394]

HEG neurofeedback is an effective training method useful for many conditions that respond to the activation of the brain's surface, or cortex. The frontal lobes, which are commonly referred to as the executive brain, are uniquely addressed using HEG. Executive

---

[392] Carman, J. A. (2004) Passive infrared hemoencephalography: Four years and 100 migraines. *Journal of Neurotherapy, 8* (3), 23-51. Retrieved from:
http://www.haworthpress.com/store/toc/J184v08n03_TOC.pdf
[393] Toomim, H., & Toomim, M. (1999) Clinical observations with brain blood flow biofeedback — the Thinking Cap™. *Journal of Neurotherapy, 3*(4),73. Retrieved from:
http://www.isnr.org/uploads/1999%20Toomim%20_%20Toomim.pdf
[394] Toomim, H., & Toomim, M. (1999) Clinical observations with brain blood flow biofeedback — the Thinking Cap™. *Journal of Neurotherapy, 3*(4),73. Retrieved from:
http://www.isnr.org/uploads/1999%20Toomim%20_%20Toomim.pdf

brain simply indicates that this portion of the brain is the executive, or director, that instructs other parts of the brain to act during conscious action. If you intend to grasp a baseball and throw it over the plate, it is the executive brain that manages the process, even though many of the muscular motions may have become almost instinctive as a result of extensive practice and operant conditioning.

HEG neurofeedback uses a simple headband fitted with either an infrared thermometer (pIR or passive infrared) or an optical detector (nIR or near-infrared HEG) to measure brain activity. It has been found to enhance brain function in half the time of more traditional EEG-based systems.[395]

For any system that uses light as its detection mechanism, hair color and density is a potential problem. For sites across the forehead from temple to temple, of course, this is not an issue. For sites elsewhere on the head, it can become one. Compared to EEG, HEG is much more dependent upon a clear light path to the scalp; EEG practitioners typically scratch the scalp with a tool to achieve good electrical contact.

This is not possible with HEG. HEG practitioners may occasionally shave a tiny patch or two of hair, but since the primary responsive control sites are across the forehead, this is not typical. Although HEG works best with hypo-perfuse (low blood flow) brain areas, research has shown that it can also be effective in hyper-perfuse (high blood flow) areas. This is typical

---

[395] Toomim, H. (2004) HEG Talk 1: A conceptual introduction to HEG. Retrieved from: http://www.biocompresearch.org/heg_talk1.htm

with issues such as anxiety. Finally, HEG neurofeedback typically achieves permanent results in approximately one-half the number of sessions or less than does EEG neurofeedback.

## *NIR HEG*

nIRHEG neurofeedback is sometimes also referred to as near-infrared (nIR) Spectroscopy or functional near infrared (fNir). It measures infrared and near infrared light absorption to measure brain blood oxygen levels, and uses this information to trigger feedback to the user.[396] Optical monitoring of tissues from the near-infrared (nIR) range (700-1300 nm) was first undertaken in 1977 by F.F. Jöbsis.[397] Because there is much greater NIR translucency of skin and bone, he found it made it possible to reach brain and muscle tissue without surgical intervention. With this technique called NIR Spectrometry, he could monitor blood oxygen and blood flow easily in brain tissue.

In 1988, Britton Chance and his students at the University Of Pennsylvania School Of Medicine developed a spectroscope to measure blood flow and oxygen in the brain and wrote a white paper about its

---

[396] Izzetoglu , K., Bunce, S., Onaral, B., Pourrezaei, K. & Chance, B. (2004) Functional Optical Brain Imaging Using Near-Infrared During Cognitive Tasks. *International Journal of Human-Computer Interaction*, *17* (2), 211 – 227.
[397] Jöbsis, FF. (1977) Noninvasive, infrared monitoring of cerebral and myocardial oxygen sufficiency and circulatory parameters. *Science. 198* (4323), 1264-1267.

use.[398] In the 1990s, Dr. Hershel Toomim discovered that spectrometry was not only a way to monitor active areas of the brain to show higher oxygen density and higher than normal temperature, but it could also be used as a source for biofeedback. He knew blood carries the fuel for the brain: oxygen and glucose. When an area of the brain is more active, the brain dilates the capillaries of the area in use to bring in more blood supply. With continued use, more capillaries and more neurons as well as synaptic connections between neurons are built in that area. With this in mind he developed Hemoencephalography (HEG), as he called it, as an alternative to EEG for determining brain function by measuring the brain blood flow. HEG has been shown to be very effective and in many cases can produce a change twice as effective and fast as EEG neurofeedback.[399]

Dr. Toomim's HEG measuring device uses an optical detector on a headband using infrared and near infrared light. It shines light through the skin and skull to assess the color of brain tissue. Oxygenated arterial blood is red, deoxygenated arterial blood is more bluish. Increased demand for nutrition results in faster blood flow and redder blood in the tissue. When the probe is placed on the desired position, a display indicates the blood oxygenation in the site under the

---

[398] Chance, B., Nioka, S., Kent, J., McCully, K., Fountain, M., Greenfeld, R. & Holtom, G. (1988) Time-resolved spectroscopy of hemoglobin and myoglobin in resting and ischemic muscle. *Anal Biochem.*, 174 (2),698-707.
[399] Toomim, H., & Toomim, M. (1999) Clinical observations with brain blood flow biofeedback — the Thinking Cap™. *Journal of Neurotherapy*, 3(4),73. Retrieved from: http://www.isnr.org/uploads/1999%20Toomim%20_%20Toomim.pdf

probe in a form we can sense. With this information we can use our minds to activate the chosen bit of cortical brain tissue, thus bringing in more oxygen and changing the color.

One advantage to using HEG over EEG is that HEG is relatively insensitive to artifacts such as muscle tension or eye blinks which may interfere with EEG neurofeedback. It also does away with the sticky contact paste required for most electrodes associated with EEG neurofeedback.[400]

## PIR HEG

In 1998, Jeffrey Carman, Ph.D., developed passive infrared Hemoencephalography (pIR HEG) under the guidance of Dr. Toomim. This technology is different from nIR HEG in that the pIR HEG optical instrument is a sophisticated infrared thermometer. It measures the heat radiated from the brain when activated. Dr. Carmen's research focused on the frontal lobe activation at FpZ (the center of the forehead). He has had particular success with people who suffer from migraines. His technology increases frontal lobe activity and inhibits migraine pain.[401]

---

[400] Toomim, H. (2004) HEG Talk 1: A conceptual introduction to HEG. Retrieved from: http://www.biocompresearch.org/heg_talk1.htm
[401] Carman, J. A. (2004) Passive infrared hem encephalography: Four years and 100 migraines. *Journal of Neurotherapy, 8* (3), 23-51. Retrieved from:
http://www.haworthpress.com/store/toc/J184v08n03_TOC.pdf

## LENS Neurofeedback

LENS neurofeedback was created by Len Ochs in the 1990s. The acronym, *LENS* stand for Low Energy Neurofeedback System. Ochs' system uses EEG-driven biofeedback with a very low power electromagnetic field to carry feedback along the EEG signal wires back to the person receiving it. This system lets the EEG signals themselves control the feedback. The feedback helps the brain to be aware of its own function and do something different. According to Ochs, LENS produces a measurable change in the brainwaves without conscious effort from the individual receiving the feedback. The result is a changed brainwave state, and much greater ability for the brain to regulate itself.[402]

## Conclusion

Clinicians choose the type(s) of neurofeedback they use depending upon their training and education, experience, and, perhaps, exposure to alternative types. Many prefer EEG neurofeedback because the scientific research is much broader and its history is much longer. It also gives the clinician an easier tool for placement on the scalp where dark, tightly curled hair is an issue. We prefer to use HEG neurofeedback as it has proven to be extremely effective for our patients and can be easier, cleaner and quicker to achieve a result than with EEG.

---

[402] Larsen, S. & Hartmann, T. (2006) *The Healing Power of Neurofeedback*. Rochester, VT: The Healing Arts Press.

# CHAPTER 10
# CURRENT
# NEUROFEEDBACK
# MODELS

In the last chapter we looked at the history of biofeedback and neurofeedback. In this chapter we'll look at how neurofeedback is used in treating those with brain performance issues. Neurofeedback has become an important alternative to drugs for those with brain dysfunctions ranging from ADHD and mild cognitive impairment to anxiety/depression and more. Neurofeedback helps change the way brains operate. With this tool, we can use our own thought processes to control how our brains are working.

No matter what type of neurofeedback is used, according to Dr. Hershel Toomim, creator of nIR HEG and Jeff Carmen, creator of pIR HEG, it is important to note that a person does not directly control either brainwaves or blood oxygen. These two measurements are only data that represent the response to cellular demand. In both cases what is actually being trained is the activity of the brain cells, not the dependent variables being monitored. In other words, just increasing blood flow does not necessarily produce a benefit to the brain. But increasing the activity of brain cells in an area that had previously shown low activity is a benefit and can permanently change behavior and perceived symptoms.

## EEG NEUROFEEDBACK

Today, many neurofeedback systems are based upon EEG neurofeedback, which reward brainwave frequencies measured through gelled electrodes placed on the scalp. EEG frequencies are broadly associated with various mental states[403], as shown in Table 10-1. For example, most ADHD patients exhibit similar surface EEG disturbances. Specifically, 85-90% of patients with ADHD display signs of cortical "hypo-arousal," (or under-aroused) a parasympathetic shutdown which can look like depression, a mental "dullness" or other dissociative states found in traumatized patients.

---

[403] Friel, P.N. (2007) EEG Biofeedback in the Treatment of Attention Deficit/Hyperactivity Disorder. *Alternative Medicine Review* , *12*, 2.

| EEG Rhythms and Associated Mental States | | |
|---|---|---|
| EEG Rhythm | Frequency(Hz) | Associated Mental States |
| Delta | 1-4 | Sleep; dominant in infants |
| Theta | 5-7 | Drowsiness; "tuned-out;" inner-directed insights |
| Alpha | 8-12 | Alertness; meditation, dominant when eyes closed |
| SMR | 12-15 | Mentally alert; physically relaxed |
| Beta | 13-21 | Focused; sustained attention; problem solving |
| High Beta 2 | 18-30 | Intensity; anxiety; hyper-vigilance |
| Gamma | 38-42 | Important in learning |

**Table 10-1: EEG Rhythms and Associated Mental States**

A smaller subgroup of ADHD patients exhibits EEG patterns suggestive of "hyper-arousal" (or over-aroused). This state is identified by excessive brain activation in the amygdala and insula (a cerebral cortex structure deep within the lateral fissure between the temporal lobe, the parietal lobe and the frontal lobe) and is associated with the "fight or flight" response.

The body is so hyper-focused on the perceived threat that one's brain can't engage in higher-order thinking and this can be seen on an EEG as greater relative beta activity, decreased relative alpha activity, and decreased theta/beta power ratios diffusely across multiple cortical recording sites.[404]

Modern EEG biofeedback systems are sold by a number of manufacturers. They consist of a set of EEG sensors which are attached to the scalp with a water-based gel and a signal transducer/amplifier connected to a computer or computers with software capable of analyzing the EEG signals. These signals perform various mathematical transformations, displaying relevant signals to the patient and providing rewards or inhibitions in the form of visual and/or audio feedback. The client learns to enhance desirable EEG frequencies and to suppress undesirable frequencies at the selected scalp location(s) by being rewarded (e.g., by progress in a video game). See Figure 10-1 below for the placement of the electrodes in a standardized 10/20 placement system that uses anatomical landmarks. The "10" and "20" refer to the 10% or 20% interelectrode distance.[405]

A typical neurofeedback session involves the patient sitting in a reclining chair, watching one video display that provides video and audio feedback, while the

---

[404] Rich, B.A., Schmajuk, M., Perez-Edgar, K.E., Fox, N.A., Pine, D.S. & Leibenluft, E. (2007) Different Psychophysiological and Behavioral Responses Elicited by Frustration in Pediatric Bipolar Disorder and Severe Mood Dysregulation . *Am J Psychiatry*, 164, 309-317. doi: 10.1176/appi.ajp.164.2.309
[405] Demos, J. (2004) *Getting Started with Neurofeedback.* New York: WW Norton Company.

therapist monitors a second display that provides detailed, real-time data on the patient's EEG during the session.

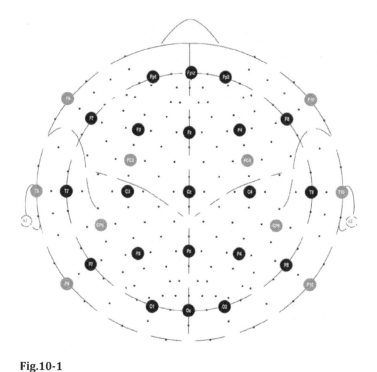

**Fig.10-1**

## ADVERSE EFFECTS OF EEG BIOFEEDBACK

Clinical researchers who have examined the effects of EEG biofeedback, in conjunction with stimulant medication, in the past have noted increased irritability, moodiness, and hyperactivity in patients who are being treated with both types of treatments concurrently.[406,407]

Other issues with using EEG neurofeedback are:

- Artifact noise which limits training to areas other than forehead for frontal lobes
- Sticky electrodes
- Typical treatment requires a 40 session minimum

## QEEG

A number of valuable imaging techniques of the brain are currently available including PET scans, functional MRI, SPECT scans, and MEG. Unfortunately, these tests can be costly and, in some cases, there are risk factors associated with the procedures. For example, a PET scan measures the metabolic activity of the brain and can be a good test for localizing areas of unusual activity within the brain. However, PET scans involve the injection of a radioactive material into the blood stream and are considered unsafe for repeated use over a short period of time or with pregnant women and small children. Similar radiation risk, pricing, and limited availability are also true of other imaging techniques such as rCBF (which measures regional cerebral blood flow), MEG (which assesses brain

---

[406] Lubar, J. F. (Ed.) (2003). Quantitative Electroencephalographic Analysis (QEEG) Databases for Neurotherapy:Description, Validation, and Application. New York: The Haworth Medical Press.
[407] Monastra, V. J. (2003). Clinical applications of electroencephalographic biofeedback. In M. S. Schwartz & F. Andrasik (Eds.), *Biofeedback: A practitioner's guide* (3rd ed., pp. 438–463). New York: Guilford Press.

electromagnetic activity), and MRS (magnetic resonance spectroscopy).[408]

A quantitative electroencephalogram (qEEG) is a special type of electroencephalogram and is often referred to as a "brain map." A brain map is used as a diagnostic tool to show brain function at a specific point in time using non-invasive means. The test has no injectable material, no side effects, can be re-administered without issues, does not require the patient to be completely still, and is safe for pregnant women and small children.

The qEEG data shows a pattern of electrical functioning of the brain in the various frequencies through computer technology. A color-coded "map" is produced to show areas of discrepancies in brain function in beta, alpha, theta and delta frequencies.[409]

A normative reference database is used to compare data retrieved from the procedure. It allows the clinician to compare results to clinically normal or otherwise healthy individuals in the same age group, gender, etc. in order to identify the measures that are deviant from normal and the magnitude of deviation. Normative databases themselves do not diagnose a patient's clinical problem. Rather, a trained professional first evaluates the patient's clinical history and clinical symptoms and complaints and then uses

---

[408] Raichle, M.E. (2003) Functional Brain Imaging and Human Brain Function. *The Journal of Neuroscience, 23* (10), 3959-3962.
[409] Pechura, C. M., & Martin, J. B. (1991) Mapping the Brain and Its Functions: Integrating Enabling Technologies Into Neuroscience Research. Institute of Medicine (U.S). Committee on a National Neural Circuitry Database.

the results of normative database comparisons in order to aid in the development of an accurate clinical diagnosis.[410]

In the 1980s and 1990s researchers such as Dr. E. Roy John at New York University Medical Center as well as Frank H. Duffy, M.D. at Harvard Medical School both published papers showing the efficacy of brain maps as a tool to measure brain function. Over the last twenty years, many more studies have concluded that brain map findings are comparable with other types of brain analysis. Moreover, with brain maps, subtle brain dysfunction can be detected that is not discernible at all with other methods.[411]

It is important to note that there is a difference between brain maps and other commonly used, and perhaps more familiar, imaging techniques. For example, x-rays, CAT scans and MRIs are all used to measure brain anatomy or structure. The brain map, on the other hand, measures brain physiology or function. It is also important to understand that a brain map-qEEG-is not the same as an EEG or EEG neurofeedback.

An EEG is used in real time to evaluate if an individual has epilepsyor to determine if there is serious brain pathology, such as a tumor. EEG neurofeedback, as we

---

[410] Demos, J. (2004) *Getting Started with Neurofeedback.* New York: WW Norton Company.
[411] Thatcher, R.W. & Lubar, J.F. (2008) History of the Scientific Standards of QEEG Normative Databases. in Budzinsky, T, Budzinski, H. ,Evans, J.& Abarnel, A. (2008)*Introduction to QEEG and Neurofeedback:Advanced Theory and Applications"*. San Diego: Academic Press.

have explained, uses the same type of brain signals as a basis to feed back stimuli to produce a certain result. A

qEEG brain map evaluates the manner in which a particular person's brain functions. It is not designed to diagnose tumors, epilepsy, or other structural medical conditions. EEG neurofeedback practitioners typically use the information garnered from a brain map to pinpoint areas on the scalp to train.

To the HEG neurofeedback practitioner, a brain map can be useful, particularly in cases of traumatic brain injury, stroke or post-traumatic stress disorder. There, too, the brain map can be a guide to training activity and to determine changes that occur over the course of treatment.

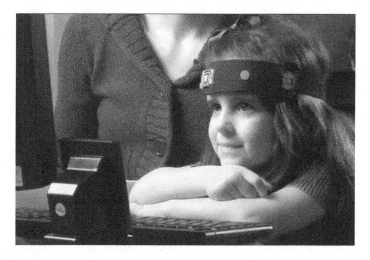

**Fig.10-2**

Since bone is translucent, the nIR HEG lights shine through the skull and through the brain tissue. The light refracts (bends) through the brain tissue and the red or infrared component of the signal is absorbed more or less depending upon the oxygen level in the blood at that point. The ratio between the level of the red and infrared light is a good indicator of relative cellular activity.

The more activated the brain, the more oxygen and glucose is demanded. The arterial system responds to supply this demand and the blood color changes to a brighter red. You can change brain activity at will by intently focusing or solving a problem. These areas also see an overall increase in temperature as the glucose converted to energy to feed the cells. As we use HEG to train the brain, the increased oxygen is measured and that information is fed back to the client via sound and video.[412]

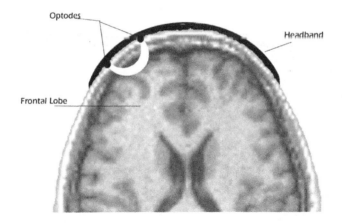

**Fig.10-3**

---

[412] Toomim, H., Mize, W., Kwong, P. C., & Toomim, M. (2004) Intentional increase of cerebral blood oxygenation using hemoencephalography (HEG). *Journal of Neurotherapy, 8* (3), 5-21. Retrieved from: http://www.biocompresearch.org/Tinius%20HEG%204%2012%2004.ht m

We use a modified version of the 10/20 electrode system with the HEG system. It is referred to as the 10/10 system as shown in Fig. 10-4. The "10" refers to the 10% inter-electrode distance. This system has more closely spaced electrodes, or in our case lights, than the standard 10/20 system. We use this system specifically because we know some of the positions not found on the 10/20 system are triggers for disorders we treat. Here is the 10/10 system:

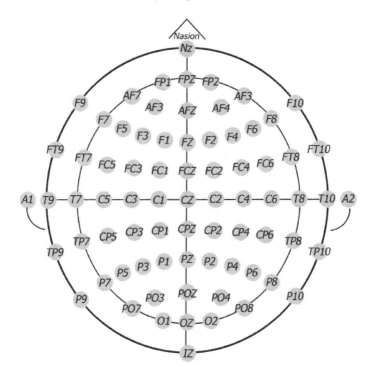

**Fig.10-4**

Passive infra-red (PIR) neurofeedback is another form of HEG developed by Jeffrey A. Carman. This form uses an infrared thermometer to measure the change in temperature brought on by activity in the brain.

Passive infra-red (PIR) neurofeedback uses an infrared thermometer to measure the change in temperature brought on by activity in the brain. This procedure is not unlike Thermography.

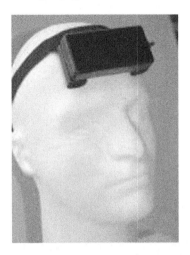

**Fig.10-5**

The PIR and the NIR types of HEG neurofeedback use slightly different wavelengths in the electromagnetic spectrum. The nIR HEG device uses a shorter wavelength than the pIR HEG device. The difference is that the longer wavelength sensor in the pIR HEG device is more sensitive to body heat. nIR HEG devices, on the other hand, are insensitive to heat in that range.

Carmen's approach to pIR HEG uses placement on the center of the forehead (fPZ) for all treatments. According to Toomim, the probable reason for this is that PIR at fPZ picks up a wide area along the prefrontal cortex and has the effect of gently increasing smooth arousal regulation. Carmen also uses an infrared camera to test pre- and post-treatment.

A positive aspect of this method is that it gives clients a visual that clearly shows changes.[413]

Both HEG techniques provide a clean, quick method that, unlike EEG neurofeedback, does not use sticky gel, abrasives and electrically sensitive electrodes. Also, the number of HEG treatment sessions is typically 10-20 sessions, rather than the 40 sessions typical with EEG neurofeedback. A huge advantage to using HEG is that it virtually eliminates noise from facial movement, which is common in EEG raw data, so training can be done where it's most useful on the frontal lobes. However, HEG is not limited to the frontal lobes; with care, it can be useful on other areas as well.

In the past those who used HEG were hampered by the idea that HEG was only useful in hypo-aroused brains. However, we have found that using trigger points and supplemental technologies, HEG has been shown effective for these issues as well.

HEG is most useful to significantly improve:

- Concentration
- Focus
- Memory
- Anxiety/depression
- Addiction
- General cognitive function
- Migraines
- ADHD/autism

---

[413] Carman, J. A. (2004) Passive infrared hemoencephalography: Four years and 100 migraines. *Journal of Neurotherapy, 8* (3), 23-51. Retrieved from:
http://www.haworthpress.com/store/toc/J184v08n03_TOC.pdf

## ADVERSE EFFECTS OF HEG BIOFEEDBACK

Adverse effects of HEG neurofeedback are few. It is non-invasive except to the extent of the beam from a single red LED in nIR HEG devices. The only side effect reported seems to occur when a brain is "over-exercised". The feeling is one of fatigue, but this passes with inactivity and leaves no permanent harm. This is usually characterized as a "heavy feeling" in the frontal lobes or lightheadedness. This is usually an exaggeration of the person's usual symptoms and generally only lasts the day of the exercise. As exercise continues, we find that patients are capable of longer and longer periods of exercise without any side effects.

Occasionally a patient will report "a headache without pain". It is generally described as a throbbing feeling. It likely represents a perception of the unfamiliar sensation of increased cerebral flow to the prefrontal cortex. This usually dissipates within one minute of training.[414]

## REBECCA'S STORY

*Rebecca is a 46-year-old medical specialist with a history of repeated head traumas occurring while racing motorcycles. She was forced to close her practice because of her inability to focus or concentrate. Her reported symptoms included insomnia, anxiety, depression, mood swings, crying, irritability, and a feeling of being easily overwhelmed.*

---

[414] Biofeedback Institute of Los Angeles (2009) Foundation HemoEncephaloGraphy (HEG)Neurofeedback Certification Course. Retrieved from: www.biocompresearch.org/Foundation-HEG.pdf

*She was not responsive to a range of psychotropic medications. Homeopathy, acupuncture, antibiotics, allergy testing, diet management and antimalarial drugs were also tried but provided no relief. She reported that Eye Movement Desensitization and Reprocessing (EMDR) had helped some, but it didn't stop her from dwelling on things, as she couldn't get out of the "loops".*

*Rebecca even had her amalgam fillings removed from her teeth, but didn't really notice a difference. Occasionally she reported that she would have fleeting moments when she felt OK, but they never lasted long. She completed two EEG-based neurofeedback programs, one consisting of 80 sessions and the other 40, with no success.*

*When Rebecca came to see us, she was taking two heavy psychotropic medications to attempt to manage her disorders. She remained anxious and was unable to stop crying. Although she was sleeping, even after a night's sleep, she would wake up tired with nausea and a headache. Her appetite was decreasing and she was losing weight. With all her problems, she was finding it increasingly difficult to converse and make decisions.*

*In our initial assessment, Rebecca's tests indicated that she had low oxygen levels in the left frontal lobe of her brain where she had suffered injury. Her cognitive and memory scores were very low as were her neuromotor skills. After the first three sessions, Rebecca reported that she had stopped crying and she was feeling better. At the 10-session assessment she had been able to wean herself from one of her primary psychotropic medications and was feeling much better than she had in a long time.*

*After 20 sessions, she had weaned herself from all other medications and was functioning very well. She was no longer depressed; she could function again in the working world. Even in the face of significant family trauma, she was able to function and not fall back into depression.*

# CHAPTER 11
# ADDITIONAL
# NEUROTHERAPY
# TECHNOLOGIES

Neurofeedback is the principal weapon used by neurotherapists against brain malfunctions, but there should be other weapons in each therapist's arsenal. In this chapter we'll look at some of the therapies that we have found to be particularly effective in our treatment of those with brain issues.

## SOUND AND LIGHT

Claudius Ptolemaeus (Ptolemy) lived in Egypt in the second century AD. A Roman citizen who wrote in Greek (the language of scholarship), he researched and wrote on astronomy, geography, astrology, and music. While he is most remembered for his now-discredited system of a geocentric solar system, he is also the spiritual father of what we now call brain wave entrainment. Ptolemy noticed that a spoked wheel turning in sunlight could evoke perceived colors and even emotions in the viewer. This phenomenon was not researched further until the 20th century. The power of sound may have been first appreciated at Jericho, but the healing power of sound was well known to the Greeks and Romans.

Today we use carefully designed light and sound tools to evoke specific responses in their recipients, even to the point of controlling the dominant frequency of brain waves.

## Audio/Visual Entrainment

The brain is an electrochemical organ. According to Rodolfo Llinás of the New York University School of Medicine "...[t]he cells in the brain, like the heart, have intrinsic rhythm. They move, they oscillate, like the waves in the ocean at a certain speed, a certain velocity, a certain frequency. Cells can have different frequencies. They can oscillate very slowly, and when that happens consciousness disappears."

Electrical activity emanating from the brain can be measured as brainwaves. Research has identified four categories of brainwaves to identify different mental states. They range from the high-amplitude, low-frequency delta to the low-amplitude, high-frequency beta.

Everyone, no matter gender or age, experiences the same characteristic brainwaves. They are:

- BETA: 13-21 cycles per second; awaking awareness, extroversion, concentration, logical thinking, and active conversation. A person making a speech, a teacher or a talk show host would all be in beta when they are engaged in their work.
- ALPHA: 8-12 cycles per second; relaxation times, non-arousal, meditation, hypnosis
- THETA: 5-7 cycles per second; day-dreaming, dreaming, creativity, meditation,

paranormal phenomena, out of body
experiences, ESP, shamanic journeys.
- DELTA: 1-4 or fewer cycles per second,
deep dreamless sleep. The frequency of the
dominant brainwave dramatically affects
how well it functions for different activities.
For example, it is almost impossible to pay
attention if the brain is producing an
abundance of low alpha or theta
brainwaves. However, it is just as difficult
to fall asleep with excess high beta
brainwaves.[415]

In 1934, E.D. Adrian and B.H.C. Mathews discovered
repetitive light stimulation. They found strobing or
"photic driving" could alter brainwaves to follow and
pulse at the same frequency as the lights.[416]

In the 1950s and 1960s, photic driving continued to be
used and became known as visual entrainment or
brainwave entrainment (BWE).[417] Throughout history,
traditional and modern cultures have also sought to
generate trance-like states using music with short,
repeated phrases and a hypnotic beat. Auditory
entrainment, or the sonic driving effect, is based on the
idea that physiological functions, such as the heartbeat

---

[415] Oken, B., & Salinsky, M. (1992) Alertness and attention: Basic
science and electrophysiologic correlates. *Journal of Clinical
Neurophysiology*, 9(4), 480-494.

[416] Adrian, E. D. & Matthews, B. H. (1934) The Interpretation of
Potential Waves in the Cortex. *The Psychological Laboratory*,
Cambridge. Retrieved from: jp.physoc.org/content/81/4/440.full.pdf

[417] Siever, D. (2002) The Rediscovery of Audio Visual Entrainment
Technology. Retrieved from: http://www.mindalive.com/2_5.htm

or brainwaves, tend to synchronize to rhythmic patterns in sound.

Today we use a combination of visual and auditory technologies to enhance brain function. This technology is non-invasive and has few side effects. Those with photic sensitivities or who are prone to photic seizures may want to discuss the use of this technology with their physician before use.

The flash of lights from eyesets combined with pulses or tones from headphones creates a very effective method to entrain brainwaves to a normal range. To produce a noticeable physiological response, the sound utilized must be of the appropriate type. Typical sounds used by audio/visual devices are binaural beats, isochronic tones or clicks. As clicks are usually more irritating to users, binaural beats or isochronic tones are usually employed.

Binaural beats are created by combining two different tones, one in each ear. For the two separate tones to be perceived as one by the brain, they must be no more than 25Hz a part.[418] The binaural beat does not occur in nature and, in fact, can only be heard with headphones as the two sounds are processed by the brain. Although binaural beat technology is widely used, research has shown that binaural beats might be of very little value, as they produce a very small response in the auditory cortex of the brain.[419]

---

[418] Siever, D. (2009) Entraining Tones and Binaural Beats. Retrieved from: www.mindalive.com/1_0/article%2011.pdf

[419] Oster, G. (1973) Auditory beats in the brain. *Scientific American*, *229*, 94-102. Available from PubMed database.

Isochronic tones are different from binaural beats, as they are the same tone evenly spaced and they cause a strong response in the auditory cortex.[198] In our experience, most individuals find the isochronic tones more pleasurable and find their hypnotic qualities make it easier to dissociate, or let their mind go with the beat.

Brainwave entrainment only occurs when a constant, repetitive stimulus of sufficient strength to "excite" the thalamus is present. The thalamus passes the stimuli onto the sensory-motor strip, the cortex in general and associated processing areas such as the visual cortex in the occipital lobes and auditory cortexes in the temporal lobes.[198]

Research has shown that audio/visual entrainment (AVE) is effective in promoting relaxation, to improving cognition, and for treating ADHD,[420] depression and anxiety.[421] Studies have also shown its efficacy for Post-Traumatic Stress Disorder (PTSD) and Obsessive Compulsive Disorder (OCD). Seasonal Affective Disorder, fibromyalgia, Chronic Fatigue Syndrome (CFS), migraine headaches, chronic pain and hypertension are also helped with AVE use.[422]

---

[420] Lubar, J. F., Bianchini, B. A., Calhoun, W. H., & Lambert, E. W. (1985) Spectral analysis of EEG differences between children with and without learning disabilities. *Journal of Learning Disabilities, 18*, 403-408.
[421] Brownbeck, T., & Mason, L. (1999) Neurotherapy in the treatment of dissociation. In J. R. Evans, & A. Arbanel. (Eds)., *Introduction to quantitative EEG and neurofeedback.* San Diego: Academic Press.
[422] Siever, D. (2002) The Rediscovery of Audio Visual Entrainment Technology. Retrieved from: http://www.mindalive.com/2_5.htm

Presently more than 70 schools are using AVE for treating children with ADHD. Michael Joyce from "A Chance to Grow" in Minneapolis, Minnesota, has been the primary proponent of using AVE for ADHD. He continues to conduct studies to help special needs children.[423]

## CRANIAL ELECTROTHERAPY STIMULATION (CES)

The idea of any kind of electrical therapy can be frightening as we envision barbaric shock therapy treatments of the past. However, there is little resemblance between CES and the painful therapy of centuries past. In fact, it is usually pain-free.

CES can come as a separate unit or as an add-on to an AVE unit. It uses mild battery-powered clip-on electrodes that attach to the ear lobes. A small current is sent across the scalp so that the most a user experiences during the therapy is a brief tingling sensation on their earlobes. But this tingling is not necessary to achieve results. In fact, most people feel nothing at all. CES is a non-drug solution for the reduction of depression and anxiety. In our experience, CES attached to an AVE unit enhances the effect of AVE and works on the endorphins. [380] After a CES session the individual is alert and relaxed. CES is also useful for those who are going through drug detoxification and withdrawal. For those seeking nothing more than a good night's sleep, it is an alternative to habit-forming

---

[423] Joyce, M., & Siever, D. (2000) Audio-visual entrainment program as a treatment for behavior disorders in a school setting. *Journal of Neurotherapy. 4 (*2), 9-15. doi:10.1300/J184v04n02_04

tranquilizers. CES has few side effects associated with its use.

Research demonstrates that CES produces a mild stimulation in the hypothalamic area of the brain, resulting in balancing neurotransmitter activity (in particular Beta Endorphin and Norepinephrine). The effects achieved are similar to that of a "jogger's high".[424]

## TDCS

Transcranial DC Stimulation (tDCS) has been used by the medical world since 43AD when Scribonius Largus, physician of the Roman Emperor Claudius, used an (electric) torpedo fish to treat gout and headache. Today scientists are finding new ways of using this simple technique to help everything from depression, anxiety, and focus to motor control, mathematical prowess[425] and even enhance insight.[426]

Doctors are experimenting with tDCS to treat severe depression and help stroke victims regain their

---

[424] Bailey, S. (1999) How micro current stimulation produces ATP -- one mechanism. *Dynamic Chiropractic* 17(18): 16, 18-19.
[425] Utz, K. S., Dimova, V., Oppenlander, K., & Kerkhoff, G. (2010) Electrified minds: Transcranial direct current stimulation (tDCS) and Galvanic Vestibular Stimulation (GVS) as methods of non-invasive brain stimulation in neuropsychology-A review of current data and future implications. *Neuropsychologia*, 48(10), 2789–2810.
[426] Chi RP, Snyder AW (2011) Facilitate Insight by Non-Invasive Brain Stimulation. PLoS ONE 6(2): e16655. doi:10.1371/journal.pone.0016655

speaking skills.[427] US Air Force researchers are using it to make people better at guiding killer drones,[428] and DARPA has found it could improve snipers' marksmanship.[429]

Different than CES, tDCS applies a small current (usually around 2mA) directly to areas needing stimulation. An Anode electrode is positioned above the region of interest (Anodal stimulation tends to enhance the activity of neurons in the region of interest), while a Cathode or Reference electrode (Cathodal stimulation tends to inhibit the activity of neurons) is attached somewhere on the opposite side of the head, arm or shoulder to complete the circuit. Either the stimulating or the reference electrode may be placed above the region of interest (to either enhance or inhibit).

> In most studies done using tDCS, the reference electrode has been placed over the contralateral orbit (above the left or right eye) to avoid negative effects from it. However, the studies never looked at the

---

[427] Fields, D. (November 25, 2011) Amping Up Brain Function: Transcranial Stimulation Shows Promise in Speeding Up Learning. *Scientific American*. Retrieved from: http://www.scientificamerican.com/article.cfm?id=amping-up-brain-function.

[428] McKinley, A., M. Weisend, L. McIntire, N. Bridges, C. M. Walters, and C. Goodyear (2011) Acceleration of air force image analyst training using transcranial direct current stimulation (tdcs). *Society for Neuroscience*. 05.12/YY47

inhibiting effects that the reference electrode might have had on the prefrontal lobe. Some recent studies and in particular a study by Nitsche,[430] show that it is better to have a small stimulating electrode and large reference electrode. This way, the current density is high under the treatment electrode and weak under the reference electrode. This arrangement allows the reference electrode to be placed most anywhere over the scalp without it affecting brain function beneath it. Most studies have used stimulation at 1 ma of current through 7cm x 7cm (49 $cm^2$ ) electrodes (There are 2.54 cm in one inch, therefore a 1" square electrode is 2.54 cm x 2.54 cm = 6.45 $cm^2$). Fregni and his group at Harvard advocate using a shoulder for the reference placement. [431]

A TDCS session is typically pain free and lasts 20-30 minutes. The effects varies depending on the area being affected, but it appears to change the baseline level of cortical excitability, and the effects can last for a few days or even be permanent.[432],[433]

[430] Nitsche, M., Doemkes, T., Antal, A., Liebatanz, N., Lang, N., Tergau, F., et al. (2007) Shaping the effects of transcranial direct current stimulation of the human motor cortex. *Journal of Neurophysiology, 97, 3109-3117*

[431] Siever, D. (2013) transCranial DC Stimulation. Retrieved from *www.mindalive.com/1_0/article%2011.pdf*

[432] Fregni F, Boggio P, Nitsche M, Bermpohl F, Antal A, Feredoes E, et al (2005) Anodal transcranial direct current stimulation of prefrontal cortex enhances working memory. *Exp Brain Res.* 166: 23-30

Several studies have been performed on the safety of tDCS and on possible side effects. These studies have resulted in clear recommendations on its safe use. There is general agreement that if recommendations concerning contraindications and stimulation parameters are followed correctly, tDCS is a well-tolerated method with minimal or no side effects. [434] [435] [436]

## SOUND THERAPY

In the late 1940s, Dr. Alfred Tomatis, a French ear, nose and throat specialist, pioneered the field of sound therapy. Dr. Tomatis discovered that he could repair the damaged hearing of opera singers and factory workers by playing the sounds they could no longer hear. He also noted that by improving the way we listen, he could dramatically improve learning, balance, coordination and posture as well as communication and creativity.[437]

[433] Liebetanz D, Fregni F, Monte-Silva K, Oliveira M, Amancio-dos-Santos A, Nitsche M, et al (2006) After-effects of transcranial direct current stimulation (tDCS) on cortical spreading depression. *Neuroscience letters*. 398: 85-90

[434] Fregni F, Thome-Souza S, Nitsche M, Freedman S, Valente K, Pascual-Leone A. A controlled clinical Trial of cathodal DC polarization in patients with refractory epilepsy. Epilepsia 2006: 47: 335-342

[435] Iyer M, Mattu U, Grafman J, Lomarev M, Sato S, Wassermann E. Safety and cognitive effect of frontal DC brain polarization in healthy individuals. Neurology 2005: 64: 872-875

[436] Nitsche M, Liebetanz D, Antal A, Lang N, Tergau F, Paulus W. Modulation of cortical excitability by weak direct current stimulation – technical, safety and functional aspects. Suppl Clin Neurophysiol 2003: 56: 255-276

[437] Tomatis, A.A. (1991) *The Conscious Ear*, Paris: Station Hill Press.

Listening is very different from hearing. Hearing is passive and automatic—we don't have to think consciously to hear a sound. However listening is an active process we can choose to do or not. Just as you can look without seeing, you can also hear without listening. Listening requires the desire to focus on sounds.

Sound itself is an interesting phenomenon because we hear with more than just our ears. Our skin and bones are also sensitive conductors. As a matter of fact, your body can pick up a sound that warns the brain milliseconds before the sound is actually heard by our ears.[438] When this happens the sound is transmitted directly to our inner ear without any filter to lessen its intensity and therefore produces a reflex reaction or a shudder. When sounds are picked up by our ears, they are filtered to a more comfortable intensity.[383]

Many people with listening issues or a poor ability to process the sounds they hear are misdiagnosed as having other problems. These auditory processing issues create poor attention and behavior, weak communication skills, a lack of body coordination, abnormal energy levels, ineffective learning abilities and faulty sensory integration. Often those with auditory processing issues are misdiagnosed as ADHD, autistic, bipolar or as having a learning disorder.[439]

---

[438] Moore, Brian C.J. (1982) An introduction to the psychology of hearing. New York, Academic Press

[439] Corbett, B. A., Shickman, K. & Ferrer, E. (2007) A brief report :The effects of Tomatis sound therapy on language in children with autism. Retrieved from: http://www.ncbi.nlm.nih.gov/pubmed/17610057

The good news is that training improves or enhances the ability to process sound. Sound therapy helps to exercise and tone the tiny muscles in the ear and helps to build stronger multi-sensory pathways in the brain. This improves the ability to process sound and enhances auditory processing skills, cognitive abilities and enhances brain function. As the ear and brain become more receptive to high frequency sounds, discrimination of tones becomes easier. It helps sequential memory difficulties, and the ability to discriminate speech against a variety of background noises so distractions by other sounds in the environment are minimized. This is especially helpful to children who have issues with attention and focus in a classroom.[440]

Sound Therapy uses specially recorded acoustically-modified music to stimulate the vestibular system in the inner ear. Through the auditory nerve the Limbic System, which is the emotional center of the brain, is stimulated to allow you to affect behavior, auditory processing, cognition and anger issues.[441] There are now many forms of sound therapy marketed under various labels:

- Auditory retraining
- Listening retraining
- Music-based auditory retraining

[440] Tomatis, A.A. (1991) *The Conscious Ear*, Paris: Station Hill Press.
[441] Harper, J. & Weiner, A. L. (2010) Reaching Combined Interventions: Effectively addressing attention and auditory- processing issues in school-aged children. *ADVANCE for Occupational Therapy Practitioners.* Retrieved from: http://occupational-therapy.advanceweb.com/ebook/magazine.aspx?EBK=OT010410#/27/

Depending upon the program design, execution, and application, sound therapy can be more or less effective. It can be surprisingly effective, however, in a well-designed program when coupled with other complementary therapies.

## NEUROMOTOR DEVELOPMENT

Parents can tell you when a child took his first step. This is a huge milestone in early childhood development. However, the sensory integration and learned motor skills that normally occur during early development leading to this milestone are the foundations for movement patterns throughout a person's life.[442] If these skills are not learned or a problem occurs with the integration and processing of information, poor motor planning and sequencing can be a life-long issue.

Neuromotor exercises are used to improve the processing abilities that are central to human activity—from the coordinated movements needed to walk or climb stairs to choosing the order of words in a sentence to provide meaning.

As you will recall, neurotransmitters are the chemicals by which neurons connect and communicate to other neurons. Acetylcholine is used in the central nervous system as a neurotransmitter involved in memory, attention, and certain other functions. In the peripheral nervous system, acetylcholine is the only

---

[442] Wiley, S. & Moeller, M.P. (2007) Disabilities In Children Who Are Deaf/Hard Of Hearing. *The ASHA Leader, 12*(1), 8-9, 28-29

neurotransmitter used to communicate to skeletal muscles.

Another of the brain's neurotransmitters, dopamine, helps regulate fine motor movement.[443] Each skeletal muscle is made up of thousands of individual muscle fibers and each of these is controlled by one alpha motor neuron in either the brain or the spinal cord. On the other hand, each single alpha motor neuron controls many muscle fibers (ranging from a few to a hundred or more), forming a functional unit referred to as a motor unit. These motor units are the critical link between the brain and muscles. The brain not only controls the actions of the motor neurons and muscles, but also the nature of the feedback that it receives from sensory receptors in the muscles as movements occur.[444]

The point at which nerves communicate with muscle tissue is called a neuromuscular junction. When acetylcholine is released at a neuromuscular junction, it crosses the tiny space (synapse) that separates the nerve from the muscle. It then binds to acetylcholine receptor molecules on the muscle fiber's surface. This initiates a chain of events that lead to muscle contraction. These neurotransmitters, then, regulate body movement and complete the intimate relationship between body and mind, muscle and memory.[390]

---

[443] Schultz W (2007) Multiple dopamine functions at different time courses. *Annu. Rev. Neurosci.* 30: 259–88. doi:10.1146/annurev.neuro.28.061604.135722
[444] Russell, Peter (2013). *Biology - Exploring the Diversity of Life*. Toronto: Nelson Education.

Scientists have shown that muscle fiber contains scaffolding made of specialized proteins that hold these acetylcholine receptors in place. In 2004, Jeff W. Lichtman, M.D., Ph.D., at Washington University School of Medicine in St. Louis, demonstrated that inactivity created a loss of nerve signals that actually disassembled this scaffolding and caused a loss of acetylcholine receptors. When the muscle became active again, however, the scaffolding once again held passing acetylcholine receptors in place. "So muscle activity signals to keep a synapse stable, and synaptic inactivity can also signal to disassemble a synapse," says Lichtman, a professor of neurobiology. "So if you lose activity, you lose receptors. But if you regain activity, you get those receptors back." [445]

Neuromotor skills training works by enhancing internal processing speed within the cerebellum, prefrontal cortex, cingulate gyrus and basal ganglia. These parts of the brain are responsible for human timing as well as other day to day functions such as sustained attention, language formulation, motor coordination and balance.[446] Neuromotor skills training has been shown to improve:

- Attention and concentration
- Motor planning and sequencing

---

[445] Akaaboune, M., Culican, S. M., Turney, S. G. & Lichtman, J. W. (1999) Rapid and Reversible Effects of Activity on Acetylcholine Receptor Density at the Neuromuscular Junction in Vivo. *Science . 286* (5439) 503 – 507. doi: 10.1126/science.286.5439.503
[446] Alpiner, N. (2004) The role of functional MRI in defining auditory-motor processing networks. *65th Annual American Physical Medicine and Rehabilitation Conference*. Retrieved from http://www.interactivemetronome.com/IMPublic/research.aspx

- Language processing
- Behavior (aggression and impulsivity)
- Balance and gait
- Endurance
- Strength
- Motor skills
- Coordination

We have used several different systems for neuromotor skills training, including one of our own design. Before their initial assessment, most patients are certain that they can perform perfectly on the relatively simple timing and sound discrimination tests we begin with. They are almost universally dismayed by their poor performances! Performance typically improves over time with repeated and diverse training. On their final assessments, patients are also typically amazed at the progress they have made.

## SENSORY INTEGRATION DEVELOPMENT

The body has five basic sensory systems. They are responsible for sight, sound, smell, taste, temperature, pain, and the position and movements of the body. The brain creates an integrated picture of the information received from each system allowing the body to make sense of its surroundings and respond appropriately. This ongoing relationship between behavior and brain functioning is called Sensory integration (SI). SI provides a crucial foundation for complex learning and behavior. Problems with sensory integration are caused from the brain's inability to integrate information received from these sensory systems.[447]

For example, those who suffer from sensory integration disorders may have trouble blocking out extraneous sounds and light. They might have vestibular issues that appear as balance and coordination deficits.[448]

The therapy for sensory integration is specific to each individual. They might be able to benefit from auditory retraining, controlled auditory and visual stimulation, cognitive or physical exercise, and neuromotor skills training to retrain the mind-body system and alleviate the symptoms.

## COGNITIVE TRAINING

Cognitive training has become a household word in the last few years. Unfortunately, not every brain activity results in improvement in brain performance. Although videogame makers such as Nintendo have tapped into this market with games such as Brain Age and Brain Age 2, Nintendo is careful to disclaim any medical value to their products. The most effective cognitive training is that which uses specific areas of the brain and trains those areas in specific ways.

For example, researchers at the Swedish medical university Karolinska Institute have shown that active

---

[447] Macaluso, E. & Driver, J. (2005) Multisensory spatial interactions: a window onto functional integration in the human brain. *Trends in Neurosciences* 28: 263–271.
[448] Kandel, E. R., Schwartz ,J.H. & Jessel, T.M. (2000) *Principles of Neural Science*. Hightstown, NJ: McGraw-Hill Professional.

training of working memory brings about visible changes in the number of dopamine receptors in the brain. The study, which was published in the February 2009 issue of *Science*,[449] used PET scans to provide deeper insight into the complex relationship between the brain's biological structure and cognition.

"Brain biochemistry doesn't just underpin our mental activity; our mental activity and thinking process can also affect the biochemistry," says Professor Torkel Klingberg, who led the study. "This hasn't been demonstrated in humans before, and opens up a floodgate of fascinating questions."[450]

Dopamine plays a key part in many of the brain's functions. Disruptions to the dopamine system can impair working memory, making it more difficult to remember information over a short period of time, such as a phone number. Impaired working memory has proved to be a contributing factor in such disorders as ADHD and schizophrenia.

Professor Klingberg and his colleagues previously demonstrated that working memory can be improved with intensive cognitive training. Now they have proven that such training actually changes the number

---

[449] McNab,F., Varrone, A., Farde,L., Jucaite, A., Bystritsky, P.,Forssberg et al (2009) Changes in Cortical Dopamine D1 Receptor Binding Associated with Cognitive Training. *Science*, 6 February 2009.

[450] McNab, F , Varrone, A., Farde, L., Jucaite, A., Bystritsky, P., Forssberg, H. & Klingberg, T. (2009) Changes in Cortical Dopamine D1 Receptor Binding Associated with Cognitive Training. *Science*, *323*(5915), 800 – 802. DOI: 10.1126/science.1166102

of dopamine D1 receptors in the cortex.[451] Our own experience has shown us that cognitive software trains those skills which allow learning to take place. Over time, as skills are exercised, the areas of the brain which are stimulated make new neural net connections making it easier to recall information. The skill set found in most software on the market target the following:[452]

- Attention
- Visual processing
- Auditory processing
- Sensory integration
- Memory and thinking skills

By itself, cognitive training is beneficial but does not typically produce significant behavioral or performance gains when used alone. When it is a part of an integrated system, however, it can add significant value.[453]

## OXYGEN THERAPIES

Oxygen therapies such as Hyperbaric Oxygen therapy (Hbot) and External Counter Pulsation (ECP) are extremely helpful to improve brain function. We use these modalities mainly for traumatic brain injury and

---

[451] McNab F, Klingberg T (2008). Prefrontal cortex and basal ganglia control access to working memory. *Nature Neuroscience*, 11(1): 103-107. doi:10.1038/nn2024.
[452] Arias-Carrión, O. & Drucker-Colín R. (2007) Neurogenesis as a therapeutic strategy to regenerate central nervous ystem. Rev Neurol 45: 739-745
[453] Klingberg, T. (2010) Training and plasticity of working memory. *Trends in Cognitive Science*,14(7): 317-324.

strokes but can be very useful in Parkinson's patients, dementia and autism. See chapter 4 for more information on these therapies.

## CATHY'S STORY

*Cathy has a history of head injury and mild depressions along with a diagnosis of Chronic Fatigue Syndrome for which she had been seeing a homeopathic doctor. Our tests revealed that she had very poor auditory processing, poor neuromotor skills, low cognitive assessment, and poor memory for phone numbers and faces. She also commented to me that she had taken Arthur Murray dance lessons but that she had no rhythm. Other patients in our office commented to us that she spoke very loudly and intrusively.*

*We treated her with sound therapy, neuromotor skills training, and HEG neurofeedback. After 10 sessions, other patients in the office remarked to us how much more quietly she spoke. She also noticed that she was remembering phone numbers and faces better. She felt much more upbeat, as well.*

*After 20 sessions, Cathy remarked that she had gone dancing and for the first time ever she was on beat with the music. Her depression was gone and her memory was noticeably better. She commented that she no longer forgot what her intentions were went she went from one room to another.*

*One year later Cathy is still improving. She says she notices every day that her hearing is better and her memory has improved.*

## REGULATING NEUROTHERAPY

Neurotherapy remains unregulated in most countries. In the US, a neurotherapy provider is not required to have a clinical license by any state or the federal government. (Regulation of health practitioners is largely a matter for the states to regulate, so the lack of any federal or national regulation is not surprising).

Moreover, many practitioners and vendors that don't follow clinical guidelines call themselves neurofeedback or brain training in part so that they do can avoid regulation. Most of these are in fact relaxation or meditation training and are bought and used by non-professionals.

Since certification is not typically required in this field, there is a wide variation in skill, knowledge, training and preparation among so-called neurotherapy practitioners. Still, there has been some attempt by private bodies to create and publish certification standards and test practitioners.

Although no certification will tell you how good your neurotherapist is at his or her job, it's important to know what certifications are acknowledged for each type of neurofeedback. For those clinicians using EEG-based equipment, there is only one certification acknowledged by most professionals. The Biofeedback Certification Institute of America (BCIA) certification "demonstrates professionalism and adherence to carefully developed standards as a health care provider. Procedures are consistent with the Department of Health & Human Services Guidelines, giving credibility and evidence that your practitioner maintains knowledge and skill levels. Health care professionals using EEG biofeedback who achieve BCIA Certification demonstrate commitment to professionalism by completing basic degree and educational requirements, learning to apply clinical biofeedback skills during mentorship, and passing a written examination."

The BCIA does not, however, certify HEG neurofeedback. The Biofeedback Institute of Los Angeles (BILA) is currently the only certifying body in the US for HEG neurofeedback. We are certified under BILA to certify others in this field.

So how and why should you choose a certified practitioner? If you want reimbursement from your insurance company, they probably will require a certified neurotherapist. Moreover, neurofeedback is not inexpensive, whether you are paying out of pocket or it's being paid for by an insurance company.

You should get the best for your money. Prospective clients should do their homework to make sure that their neurotherapist has the education they say they have. Call the certification boards and ask if the therapist is truly certified. Ask for references, look at their publication history, and speak with other people in your community. We have seen excellent practitioners in our field, but also have seen others with phony credentials and falsified records. Be careful!

# CHAPTER 12
# ATTENTION DEFICIT
# DISORDER (ADHD)

We all have difficulty at one time or other in our lives when we can't sit still, pay attention, or control impulsive behavior. However, for some children and adults this problem can be so overwhelming that it interferes with their daily lives at home, at school, at work, and in social settings. Attention-deficit/hyperactivity disorder (ADHD) is characterized by developmentally inappropriate impulsivity, inattention, and in some cases, hyperactivity. It is most often diagnosed just on observed behavior.

Parents with ADHD children can find their behaviors difficult to endure. At the same time those who are suffering with ADHD symptoms can find it is a huge blow to self-esteem. Until recently, it was believed that children outgrew ADHD in adolescence. However, it is now known that ADHD symptoms can continue into adulthood. In fact, ADHD does not develop spontaneously in adults. If you have ADHD as an adult then you had ADHD symptoms as a child even if they went undiagnosed.[454]

---

[454] Stanford, C. & Tannock, R. (29 February 2012). Behavioral Neurobiology of Attention Deficit Hyperactivity Disorder and Its Treatment. *Springer*. pp. 10–.

---

During childhood, the condition is more common in boys than girls, but this ratio appears to even out by adulthood. Adults with ADHD may be chronically late to work or to important events. They may be disorganized, restless, and have difficulty relaxing. Some people with ADHD have trouble concentrating while reading. Mood swings, low self-esteem, and poor anger management are also common problems.

It is often hard to estimate the number of adults with ADHD as often adults tend to self-medicate to minimize their symptoms with caffeine, alcohol, drugs and nicotine. Although individuals with ADHD can be very successful in life, if the disorder goes undiagnosed or untreated, they may struggle at work and in relationships, and have chronic emotional difficulties such as anxiety and depression.[455]

## LISA'S STORY

*Lisa was 11 years old. She had very few friends and fought daily with her family and peers. She was doing poorly in class. When things didn't go perfectly, she would melt down and cry. She had difficulty staying on task and wasn't turning in her homework even though many times her parents had watched her finish it.*

*Her parents began to worry. Her sleep was starting to be affected. She had only deprecating things to say about herself and she was becoming more and more angry and withdrawn. Lisa's teacher told her parents that Lisa had*

---

[455] Stanford, C. & Tannock, R. (29 February 2012). Behavioral Neurobiology of Attention Deficit Hyperactivity Disorder and Its Treatment. *Springer*. pp. 10–.

*ADHD and that should see the school psychiatrist. The psychiatrist had told them there were no good alternatives to medication. Neurotherapy, he said, was only experimental and there was no "real" proof that it worked. Attention deficit drugs were their only option.*

*Fortunately for Lisa, her parents were not convinced that drugs were the only option. They had researched the attention deficit drugs and knew that they carried a black box warning from the FDA because of their serious and potentially fatal side effects. They were unwilling to subject their daughter's health to these drugs. While researching ADHD, they read numerous reports on the effectiveness of neurotherapy and brought her to us at BrainAdvantage for assessment and training.*

*After extensive assessments, no issues with attention issues were found at all! What we did find was that her brain oxygen levels were quite low in the right frontal lobe. She was unable to utilize the oxygen as well as she could on the left. She was over-sensitive to sound and light as well, which made it very difficult for her to concentrate in class. Any extraneous sound would grab her attention, making it hard to listen only to the teacher's voice.*

*She was allergic to glutens and caseins and showed signs of depression. Her amygdala in the limbic system, the emotional center of the brain, was being over-stimulated while the frontal lobes that are used for attention, focus and memory were under-stimulated making it very hard for Lisa to stay on task.*

*After a half-dozen sessions of BrainAdvantage training, her mother commented that the principle thing she noticed about Lisa was that there was a "loss of drama". By the tenth session, she was doing markedly better in school. Her sister was starting to struggle in her attempts to maintain control of Lisa as she couldn't "press her buttons" any more.*

Lisa also began reacting quite differently to situations. By the twentieth session, Lisa was a happy, confident little girl with new friends and activities. She proudly announced she was "the third-smartest 2nd grader in her school". She also offered that this was the "start of her new life".

## ADHD CAUSES

Attention Deficit/Hyperactivity Disorder is not like other illnesses where you can observe a measurable rise in temperature or a see a visible skin rash. ADHD is a collection of behavioral symptoms, not all of which affect each ADHD individual. Because of this, there are several subtypes of ADHD. In addition, different areas of the brain are affected.

Previously, an ADHD diagnosis was typically based on a series of inattention and hyperactivity symptoms outlined in the *Diagnostic & Statistical Manual for Mental Disorders, now in its 5th edition* (called the *DSM-V*). For someone to be diagnosed with ADHD, there must be a pattern of behavior, present in multiple settings (e.g., school and home), that can result in performance issues in social, educational, or work settings.

Inattention symptoms of ADHD include:

- Not paying attention to detail
- Making careless mistakes
- Failing to pay attention and keep on task
- Not listening
- Being unable to follow or understand instructions
- Avoiding tasks that involve effort
- Being distracted or forgetful
- Losing things that are needed to complete tasks

Hyperactivity-impulsivity symptoms of ADHD include:

- Fidgeting
- Squirming
- Getting up often when seated
- Running or climbing at inappropriate times
- Having trouble playing quietly
- Talking excessively or out of turn
- Interrupting

Based on these criteria, the DSM-V identifies three subtypes of ADHD:

1. ADHD, Combined Type: Both inattention and hyperactivity -impulsivity symptoms.
2. ADHD, Predominantly Inattentive Type: Inattention but not hyperactivity-impulsivity symptoms.
3. ADHD, Predominantly Hyperactive-Impulsive Type: Hyperactivity -impulsivity but not inattention symptoms.

However, some of the requirements for ADHD have changed. According to the American Psychiatric Association (APA), publisher of the latest version of the DSM, (DSM-5), the working groups decided to eliminate the DSM-IV chapter that included all diagnoses usually first made in infancy, childhood, or adolescence. Therefore ADHD was moved to the "Neurodevelopmental Disorders" chapter to reflect brain developmental correlates with ADHD."

The latest changes made for ADHD diagnosis in DSM-5 are as follows:

- Examples have been added to the criterion items to facilitate application across the life span
- The cross-situational requirement has been strengthened to "several" symptoms in each setting
- The onset criterion has been changed from "symptoms that caused impairment were present before age 7 years" to "several inattentive or hyperactive-impulsive symptoms were present prior to age 12"
- Subtypes have been replaced with presentation specifiers that map directly to the prior subtypes
- A co-morbid diagnosis with autism spectrum disorder is now allowed
- A symptom threshold change has been made for adults, to reflect their substantial evidence of clinically significant ADHD impairment. For an adult diagnosis to be made, the patient only needs to meet five symptoms — instead of six required for younger persons — in

either of the two major domains: inattention
and hyperactivity/impulsivity [456],[457],[458],[459]

## ADHD AND THE BRAIN

In the last two decades, much more information has
been discovered about brain function and how it differs
in ADHD diagnosed individuals. With the help of new
imaging techniques the function of the brain can be
observed as well as its anatomy. Functional magnetic
resonance imaging (fMRI), magnetoencephalography,
Functional Near Infrared Spectroscopy (fNIRS),
positron emission tomography (PET), and single
photon emission computed tomography (SPECT) and
qualitative electroencephalogram (qEEG) can all
measure the changes in brain activity.

---

[456] American Psychiatric Association (2013) DSM-5 Implementation
and Support. Retrieved from
http://www.dsm5.org/Pages/Default.aspx
[457] Kieling, C., Kieling, R.R., Frick, P.J., Rohde, L.A., Moffitt, T., Nigg, J.T.,
et al (2010) The age at onset of attention deficit hyperactivity disorder.
American Journal of Psychiatry, 2010; 167:14-15.
[458] Kraemer, H.K., Shrout, P.E. & Rubio-Stipec, M. (2007) Developing
the Diagnostic and Statistical Manual V: what will "statistical" mean in
DSM-V? Social Psychiatry & Psychiatric Epidemiology, 2007; 42: 259-
267.
[459] Kuhl, E.A., Kupfer, D.J. & Regier, D.A. (2011) Patient-centered
revisions to the DSM-5. *Virtual Mentor*, 2011; 13: 873-879.

---

Areas of the brain which are commonly identified as being affected by ADHD are:

- **The frontal lobes** which help us to pay attention to tasks, focus concentration, make good decisions, plan ahead, learn and remember what we have learned. The frontal lobes also help us to behave appropriately for a given situation. Emotional issues such as anger, frustration, and irritability that come on impulsively in some types of ADHD probably come from the pre-frontal cortex. Functional imaging scans show us that the frontal cortical regions of the brain are critical to executive function, impulsivity, attention and focus. A wide selection of abnormalities in brain structure in ADHD has been reported including decreased overall cerebral tissue volume in the prefrontal region or its asymmetry.
- **The inhibitory mechanisms of the cortex** which keep us from being hyperactive, from saying things out of turn, or from getting mad at inappropriate times. These inhibitory mechanisms of the cortex help us to "inhibit" our behaviors. It has been said that 70% of the brain is there to inhibit the other 30% of the brain. When the inhibitory mechanisms of the brain aren't working efficiently, impulsive behaviors, quick temper, poor decision making and hyperactivity are apparent.
- **The Limbic System** is the core of our emotions. If the limbic system is over-activated, a person might have wide mood swings, or quick temper outbursts. He might also be "over-aroused," quick to startle, touching everything around him and hyper-vigilant.

A normally functioning limbic system would provide for normal emotional changes, normal levels of energy, normal sleep routines, and normal levels of coping with stress. A dysfunctional limbic system results in problems in all those areas. Various studies report atrophy in the corpus callosum or caudate nucleus [460],[461],[462],[463] as well as decreased volumes in the right globus pallidus, and right anterior frontal region. Functional imaging studies have suggested particular disruption of frontal-striatal and frontal-parietal circuitry.[464]

---

[460] Castellanos, F. X., Lee, P. P., Sharp, W. S., Jeffries, N. O., Greenstein, D. K. et al. (2002) Developmental trajectories of brain volume abnormalities in children and adolescents with Attention-Deficit/Hyperactivity Disorder. *Journal of the American Medical Association, 288,* 1740-1748. Retrieved from: http://jama.ama-assn.org/cgi/content/abstract/288/14/1740

[461] Sowell, E. R., Thompson, P.M., Welcome, S. E., Henkenius, A. L., Toga, A.W. & Peterson, B.S. (2003) Cortical abnormalities in children and adolescents with attention-deficit hyperactivity disorder. Lancet , 362,1699–707.

[462] Mackie, S., Shaw, P., Lenroot, R., Pierson, R., Greenstein, D.K. et al. (2007) Cerebellar development and clinical outcome in attention deficit hyperactivity disorder. *Am J Psychiatry 164,* 647–55.

[463] Shaw P, Lerch J, Greenstein D, Sharp W, Clasen L, Evans A, et al. (2006) Longitudinal mapping of cortical thickness and clinical outcome in children and adolescents with attention-deficit/hyperactivity disorder. *Arch Gen Psychiatry. 63* (5), 540-9.

[464] Dickerson, S. S. & Kemeny, M. E. (2004) Acute stressors and cortisol responses: A theoretical integration and synthesis of laboratory research. *Psychol. Bull, 130,* 355–391.

---

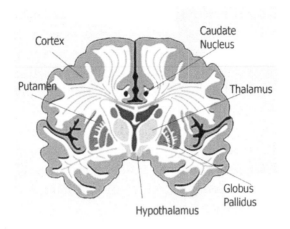

Cortex

Caudate
Nucleus

Putamen

Thalamus

Globus
Pallidus

Hypothalamus

**Fig.12-1**

- **Cerebellum** is the hind brain. It controls our
  balance and postural stability, and is involved in
  motor coordination, however, not in the initial
  learning of motor skills, but in the performance and
  improvement of learned motor skills. The
  hindbrain, although far from the frontal lobes, is
  connected to this region, most especially through
  the pons and the thalamus. Recent rat studies have
  also suggested that the cerebellum may be involved
  in some way in remembering strong emotions, and
  in the consolidation of long-term memories of fear.
  There is also growing evidence that the cerebellum
  might also be involved in processing speech and
  language.[465]

---

[465] Llinas, R.R. (2011) Cerebellar motor learning versus cerebellar
motor timing: the climbing fibre story. *The Journal of physiology* 589:
3423-3432.

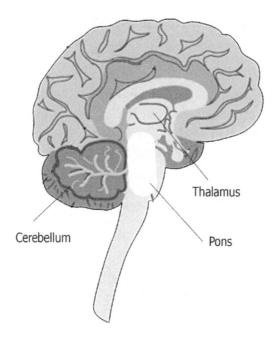

Thalamus

Cerebellum

Pons

**Fig.12-2**

- **The Reticular Activating System (RAS)** is the attention center of the brain. It is the key to "turning on your brain," and is also the center of motivation.

The Reticular Activating System is connected at its base to the spinal cord where it receives information directly from the ascending sensory tracts. The brain stem reticular formation runs all the way up to the mid-brain. To understand more fully what the RAS does, imagine that you're walking through a busy shopping mall. Think of all the noise—hundreds of people talking, music and announcements. How much of this noise is brought to your attention? Not a lot. True, you can hear a general background noise, but most of us don't bother to listen to each individual sound. [466]

But then a new announcement comes over the public address system—saying your name. Suddenly your attention is focused. Your RAS is the automatic mechanism inside your brain that brings relevant information to your attention.

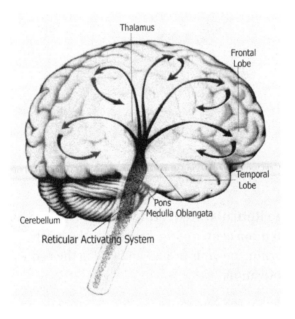

Fig.12-3

Your reticular activating system is like a filter between your conscious mind and your subconscious mind. It takes instructions from your conscious mind and passes them on to your subconscious. For example, the

[466] Evans, B.M. (2003) Sleep, consciousness and the spontaneous and evoked electrical activity of the brain. Is there a cortical integrating mechanism?. *Neuophysiologie clinique* 33: 1–10.

instruction might be, "listen for anyone saying my name." For this reason the RAS plays an important role in learning and memory. It determines impulsivity and motor activity levels which allow a person to be highly motivated or bored. When functioning normally, it provides the neural connections that are needed for the processing and learning of information, and the ability to pay attention to the correct task. If the RAS is not functioning adequately, the neurons of the cortex are under-aroused. This causes difficulty in learning, little self-control and poor memory. In fact, if the RAS failed to activate the cortex at all, one would see a lack of consciousness or even coma. On the other hand, if the RAS is too excited, the neurons of the cortex are over-aroused. In this event we see individuals with excessive startle responses, hyper-vigilance, touching everything, talking too much, restless, and hyperactive. So the RAS must be functioning normally for the rest of the brain to perform as it should.[467]

## NEUROTRANSMITTERS, BDNF AND OTHER ISSUES

Besides brain structures, neurotransmitters can play key roles in maintaining normal attentiveness and behavior. Epinephrine and norepinephrine enhance memory formation.[468] Neurotransmitter imbalances

---

[467] Evans, B.M. (2003) Sleep, consciousness and the spontaneous and evoked electrical activity of the brain. Is there a cortical integrating mechanism?. *Neuophysiologie clinique* 33: 1–10.

[468] Berridge, C. W. & Waterhouse, B. D. (2003) The locus coeruleus-noradrenergic system: modulation of behavioral state and state-dependent cognitive processes. *Brain Res.Brain Res. Rev. 42* (1), 33-84. PMID: 12668290.

have been linked to lack of focus, poor concentration, hyperactivity, and irregular sleep patterns.[469]

Norepinephrine is normally involved in vigilance and wakefulness; however, high levels of norepinephrine can reduce the rate of information processing and reduce attentiveness. One-third of the neurotransmitters in the brain are glutamate, and brain research is now looking at the intricate relationships between glutamate, dopamine, and norepinephrine in the functioning of the pre-frontal cortex.[470]

Glutamine is the pre-curser of glutamate. Dopamine and norepinephrine enhance the glutamate network neurotransmissions from the pre-frontal cortex to other areas of the brain. Too little dopamine or norepinephrine is a problem, as is too much. Although the importance of glutamate in PFC functioning is recognized in research, new findings show that neurotransmitters might not be the only issue.

Brain-derived neurotropic factor (BDNF) is a neurotrophin which enhances survival- and growth promoting activity in neuronal cells. BDNF is found in both human serum and plasma. Human platelets contain a large amount of BDNF in blood. Recent

---

[469] Bloom, B., Dey, A. N., & Freeman, G. (2006) Summary health statistics for U.S. children: National Health Interview Survey, 2005. (2006) *Vital Health Stat*.10. (231): 1-84.
[470] Tanaka M, et al. (2000) Noradrenaline systems in the hypothalamus, amygdala and locus coeruleus are involved in the provocation of anxiety: basic studies. *Eur Journal of Pharmacology*. Volume 405, Issues 1–3, 29 September 2000, Pages 397–406doi:10.1016/S0014-2999(00)00569-0

reports have suggested an impaired regulation of BDNF could be a factor in ADHD.[471] BDNF is involved in cellular plasticity, which triggers the capacity for learning and memory. Brain regions where plasticity is particularly important include the hippocampus and cortex. These are critical centers for learning and memory. The hippocampus is a central component for encoding new information, and damage there severely impairs learning. Decreased BDNF has been associated with depression, memory and cognitive deficits as well as an increased susceptibility for psychiatric disorders particularly those with a neurodevelopmental origin. Researchers at Soonchunhyang University Cheonan Hospital,[472]

South Korea found increased blood plasma levels of BDNF in untreated ADHD patients, and that plasma BDNF levels had a significant positive correlation with the severity of inattention symptoms.[473] Although neurotransmitter and BDNF imbalances are part of the puzzle, neuroscience is beginning to look at the whole picture and is moving toward a better understanding of the brain as a network, and a network of relationships.

---

[471] Tsai , S. (2009) Increased central brain-derived neurotrophic factor activity could be a risk factor for substance abuse: Implications for treatment. *Medical Hypotheses, 68* (2), 410-414.

[472] Robinson, R.C., Radziejewski, C., Stuart, D.I. & Jones, E.Y. (April 1995) Structure of the brain-derived neurotrophic factor/neurotrophin 3 heterodimer. *Biochemistry* **34** (13): 4139–46. doi:10.1021/bi00013a001

[473] Kim, J.M., Stewart, R., Kim, S.W., Yang, S..J, Shin, I.S., Kim, Y.H. et al (2008) BDNF genotype potentially modifying the association between incident stroke and depression. *Neurobiol Aging* 2008; 29: 789-792.

## Brain Networks

When we learn new things, our neurons make new connections with neighboring neurons to form neural networks. These networks reorganize and reinforce themselves in response to new stimuli. A healthy network can comprise tens of thousands of neurons totaling more than 100 trillion connections—each capable of performing 200 calculations per second! This is the structural basis of the brain's memory capacity and thinking ability.

Learning and memory involve changes to the neuron-to-neuron synapse. These are called long-term Potentiation (LTP). LTP makes communication easier between neurons, also making it easier to form memories. This creation of memories and connections within the neural networks can also be reversed. When we stop using the information stored in the network, connections begin to be lost. It is a constant process of remodeling where some connections are gained while others are lost.

According to Yi Zuo assistant professor of molecular, cell and developmental biology at the University of California, Santa Cruz, motor learning or "learning-by-doing" has been demonstrated to make a permanent mark on the brain's neural network.[474] According to Zuo, "When you learn to ride a bicycle, once the motor memory is formed, you don't forget. The same is true when a mouse learns a new motor skill; the animal

---

[474] Zuo, Y, et al. (2009) Study shows new brain connections form rapidly during motor learning. Retrieved from: www.physorg.com/news178725126.html

learns how to do it and never forgets." This is important information to understand how the brain functions to improve new learning and memory.

Recently, researchers at the University of California, Davis Center for Mind and Brain discovered that when ADHD children attempted a simple task that measured attention, two brain areas failed to connect.[475] Brain electrical rhythms were measured, in particular alpha rhythms. According to Ali Mazaheri, a postdoctoral researcher at the university, "When part of the brain is emitting alpha rhythms, it shows that it is disengaged from the rest of the brain and not receiving or processing information optimally."

The tests utilized visual or auditory cues. The child responded to cues by pressing a button. They were alerted before the tests began as to which type of cue they would be receiving. The researchers hypothesized that when visual cues were given the brain would alert the visual cortex to pay attention and a drop in alpha wave activity would occur. This was precisely what they found in non-ADHD children. However the ADHD children's brains worked differently when preparing to attend to upcoming stimuli. Their brains showed no drop in alpha wave activity indicating disconnect between the center of the brain that allocates attention and the visual processing regions.

---

[475] University of California—Davis (2010) Disconnect between brain regions in ADHD. *ScienceDaily*. Retrieved February 26, 2010, retrieved from: http://www.sciencedaily.com /releases/2010/01/100111155116.htm

Although ADHD children did improve their reaction times with practice, they didn't allocate resources as efficiently as those without ADHD. This study provides proof of a functional disconnect in ADHD brains which can be seen, giving us an opportunity to define ADHD visual data rather than just observed behavior.[476]

Another study by Spanish researchers at the Universitat Autonoma de Barcelona and the Vall de' Hebron University Hospital[477] have also found that a link exists between ADHD and the reward system in the brain. They found the ventral striatum (the major input station of the basal ganglia including the nucleus accumbens which maintains levels of motivation to complete a task) was smaller on the right side. This anomaly is associated with hyperactivity and impulsivity. The researchers concluded that ADHD is not only caused by brain alterations that affect cognitive processes, but also by brain irregularities that cause problems with motivation.

## ADHD vs. Gifted

It is common that children and adults who are affected by ADHD are quite bright.[478] Children with ADHD become bored quickly, can't sit still, and are always

---

[476] Zuo, Y, et al. (2009) Study shows new brain connections form rapidly during motor learning. Retrieved from: www.physorg.com/news178725126.html

[477] Carmona, S. et al .(2009) Ventro-Striatal reductions underpin symptoms of Hyperactivity and impulsivity in Attention-Deficit/Hyperactivity disorder. *Biol. Psychiatry, 66,* 972-977.

[478] Hodgkins P, Arnold LE, Shaw M, *et al.* (2011) A systematic review of global publication trends regarding long-term outcomes of ADHD". *Front Psychiatry* 2: 84. doi:10.3389/fpsyt.2011.00084

moving. They often act first without thinking. These actions are commonly diagnosed as ADHD. However, the same actions and behaviors can be seen with those extremely bright children who are not being challenged enough by school or their environment.

In some instances children are both ADHD and gifted. In these cases they are referred to as "Twice-Gifted" or "Twice-Exceptional." These children have unique problems. High intellect can cause ADHD to go undiagnosed. The ADHD too can cause giftedness to go unnoticed. The following chart compares behavioral issues for those with ADHD and those who are gifted but bored.

| Gifted/bored students | Students with ADHD |
|---|---|
| Poor attention and daydreaming when bored | Poorly sustained attention |
| Low tolerance for persistence on tasks that seem irrelevant to them | Diminished persistence on tasks not having immediate consequences |
| Begin many projects, see few to completion | Often shift from one uncompleted activity to another |
| Development of judgment lags behind intellectual growth | Impulsivity, poor delay of gratification |
| Intensity may lead to power struggles with authorities | Impaired adherence to commands to regulate or inhibit behavior in social contexts |
| High activity level; may need less sleep | More active, restless than other children |

| | |
|---|---|
| Difficulty restraining desire to talk; may be disruptive | Often talk excessively, often interrupt or intrude on others (e.g., butt into games) |
| Question rules, customs, and traditions | Difficulty adhering to rules and regulations |
| Lose work, forget homework, are disorganized | Often lose things necessary for tasks or activities at home or school |
| May appear careless | May appear inattentive to details |
| Highly sensitive to criticism | Highly sensitive to criticism |
| Does not exhibit problem behaviors in all situations | Problem behaviors exist in all settings, but in some are more severe |
| More consistent levels of performance at a fairly consistent pace | Used to accomplish tasks. Variability in task performance and time |

You can see by the chart that differentiating ADHD from giftedness can be difficult. Research has found two things that are useful when trying to identify one from the other.[479,480,481,482,483]

[479] Kalbfleisch, M. L. (2000) Electroencephalographic differences between males with and without ADHD with average and high aptitude during task transitions. Charlottesville: Unpublished doctoral dissertation, University of Virginia .

[480] Kaufmann, F., Kalbfleisch, M. L., & Castellanos, F. X. (2000) Attention deficit disorders and gifted students: What do we really know? *Storrs, CT*: National Research Center on the Gifted and Talented, University of Connecticut.

1.  Gifted ADHD children are more impaired than other ADHD children, suggesting the possibility that we are missing gifted children with milder forms of ADHD.
2.  High ability can mask ADHD, and attention deficits and impulsivity tend to depress the test scores as well as the high academic performance that many schools rely on to identify giftedness. Also, teachers may tend to focus on the disruptive behaviors of gifted ADHD students and fail to see indicators of high ability. Gifted children whose attention deficits are identified later may be at risk for developing learned helplessness and chronic underachievement.[484] These researchers recommend that children who fail to meet test score criteria for giftedness and are later diagnosed with ADHD be retested for the gifted program.[485],[486]

---

[481] Moon, S. M., Zentall, S. S., Grskovic, J. A., Hall, A. & Stormont, M. (2001) Emotional, social, and family characteristics of boys with ADHD and giftedness: A comparative case study. *Journal for the Education of the Gifted, 24,*207-247.

[482] Moon, S. (2002) Gifted children with attention deficit/hyperactivity disorder. In M. Neihart, S. Reis, N. Robinson, S. Moon (Eds).. *The social and emotional development of gifted children: What do we know?* (pp. 193-204). Waco, TX : Prufrock Press.

[483] Zentall, S.S., Moon, S.M., Hall, A.M., & Grskovic, J.A. (2001) Learning and motivational characteristics of boys with ADHD and/or giftedness. *Exceptional Children, 67,* 499-519.

[484] Moon, S. M., Zentall, S. S., Grskovic, J. A., Hall, A. & Stormont, M. (2001) Emotional, social, and family characteristics of boys with ADHD and giftedness: A comparative case study. *Journal for the Education of the Gifted, 24,*207-247.

[485] Baum, S.M., Olenchak, F.R., & Owen, S.V. (1998). Gifted students with attention deficits: Fact and/or fiction? Or, can we see the forest for the trees? *Gifted Child Quarterly, 42,* 96-104.

As a group, ADHD children tend to lag two to three years behind their peers in social and emotional maturity.[487] Gifted ADHD children are no exception. [488], [489] This finding has important implications for educational placement. As a group, gifted children without ADHD tend to be more similar in their cognitive, social, and emotional development to children two to four years older than children their own age.[490]

When placed with other high ability children without the disorder, ADHD children may find the advanced maturity of their classmates a challenge. Also, gifted children without the disorder may have little patience for the social and emotional immaturity of the gifted ADHD student in their midst. This is not to say that gifted ADHD students should not be placed with other gifted students. The research is clear that lack of intellectual challenge and little access to others with

---

[486] Moon, S. (2002) Gifted children with attention deficit/hyperactivity disorder. In M. Neihart, S. Reis, N. Robinson, S. Moon (Eds).. *The social and emotional development of gifted children: What do we know?* (pp. 193-204). Waco, TX : Prufrock Press.

[487] Barkley, R.A. (1998) Attention deficit hyperactivity disorder: A handbook for diagnosis and treatment. (2nd ed.). New York: Guilford.

[488] Kaufmann, F., Kalbfleisch, M. L., & Castellanos, F. X. (2000) Attention deficit disorders and gifted students: What do we really know? *Storrs, CT*: National Research Center on the Gifted and Talented, University of Connecticut.

[489] Moon, S.M., Zentall, S.S., Grskovic, J.A., Hall, A. & Stormont, M. (2001) Emotional, social, and family characteristics of boys with ADHD and giftedness: A comparative case study. Journal for the Education of the Gifted, 24,207-247.

[490] Neihart, M., Reis, S., Robinson, N., & Moon, S. (Eds.) (2002) *The social and emotional development of gifted children: What do we know?* Waco, TX: Prufrock Press.

302

similar interests, ability, and drive are o ten risk factors for gifted children contributing to social or emotional problems.

## LEARNED HELPLESSNESS

Learned helplessness is a strategy or survival technique that many individuals acquire through a childhood of failing to live up to their potential, at work, at home, and in their personal relationships. They have always failed in the past and assume they will continue to fail in the future. This is probably the biggest reason that those with ADHD are three times more likely to be depressed than their non-ADHD peers.

Research shows that children with ADHD attribute their failures or success differently than their non-ADHD peers, and that these attributions may interfere with their classroom performance. Studies have suggested the following about academic achievement and self-concept attributions of learning disabled students:

1.  Students with learning disabilities are more likely to attribute their success or failure to an outside source than their non-ADHD peers. Specifically, they are less likely to attribute success to their own ability and are more likely to attribute success to luck or external, uncontrollable and unstable factors.

2. Students with ADHD have lower self -
   esteem than non-ADHD peers.[491] This
   lowered self-esteem has been reported as
   early as grade three, and found to remain
   stable through high school. Students with
   ADHD who were neither identified nor
   given special placement experienced lower
   academic self-esteem than those who were
   identified and specifically placed. Severely
   learning disabled students who received
   full-time special placement experienced
   increased academic self-concept, especially
   in reading.[492]

## HEREDITY AND ADHD

We've seen over and over that those who have
attention deficit issues seem to have children with the
same problems. However, the strongest evidence for a
genetic link to ADHD comes from detailed studies of
twins and children who were adopted but whose
'natural' families and siblings could be traced and
investigated.[493]

---

[491] Bagwell, C. L., Molina, B., Pelham, W. E., & Hoza, B. (2001)
Attention-deficit hyperactivity disorder and problems in peer relations:
predictions from childhood to adolescence. *Journal of the American
Academy of Child and Adolescent Psychiatry, 40,* 1285-1292.
[492] Barkley, R. A. (2005) Attention deficit hyperactivity disorder: A
handbook for diagnosis and treatment (3rd ed.). New York:
Guilford.Barkley, R. A. (2011a). The Barkley Deficits in Executive
Functioning Scale. New York: Guilford Press.
[493] Sprich, S., Biederman, J., Crawford, M.H., Mundy, E., & Faraone,
S.V. (2000) Adoptive and biological families of children and
adolescents with ADHD. *J AmAcad Child Adolesc Psychiatry*
39:1432–1437.DOI: 10.1097/01.CHI.0000024883.60748.E3

One group of studies looked at the genetics and behavioral traits of both identical and non-identical twins.[494] A second group looked at adopted children and their 'natural' genetically related siblings, as well as the siblings from the adoptive families.

When researchers looked at identical twins with one twin diagnosed with ADHD, they found that there was a 72 to 83 per cent probability that the other twin would also have ADHD symptoms. This was true even where twins had been adopted and placed in different families.[495]

However, when the researchers looked at non-identical twins of the same sex, they found that the probability that both twins would have an attention deficit disorder was reduced to between 21 and 45 per cent. When researchers included the extended families of ADHD sufferers, they found that parents, siblings and children of people with attention deficit disorders were five times more likely to have the disorder than individuals who were not related to a diagnosed sufferer.

Also, strong evidence of a genetic involvement in ADHD comes from a study which found that children of

---

[494] Willcutt, E.G., Pennington, B.F., Chhabildas, N.A., Friedman, M.C. & Alexander, J. (1999) Psychiatric Comorbidity Associated With DSM-IV ADHD in a Nonreferred Sample of Twins. *Journal of the American Academy of Child; Adolescent Psychiatry.* Volume 38, Issue 11, November 1999, Pages 1355–1362

[495] Levy, F., Hay, D. A. , McStephen, M., Wood, C., et al. (1997) Attention-Deficit Hyperactivity Disorder: A Category or a Continuum? Genetic Analysis of a Large-Scale Twin Study.*Journal of the American Academy of Child & Adolescent Psychiatry: 36(6),* 737-744.

parents with the disorder had a one in two chance of having the condition themselves. For many years physicians and psychologists believed poor parenting was the cause of ADHD, today we know that poor parenting skills or poor management of an ADHD child can exacerbate the problems but they are not the primary cause of the disorder.[496]

## STREP AND ADHD SYMPTOMS

New research has shown a link between Streptococcus, or strep infections and ADHD. Pediatric Autoimmune Neuropsychiatric Disorder Associated with Streptococcus, also known as PANDAS, is a condition that leads to autoimmune-mediated inflammation of the brain,[497] and usually occurs after several bouts of Strep throat. However, ADHD symptoms may manifest even if the parent cannot recall a history of Streptococcal infection in their child. PANDAS attack a part of the brain known as the basal ganglia. The basal ganglia link the cerebral cortex (involved in rational, calm behavior) with the primitive areas of the brain (involved in fear, anger, and uncontrolled emotion). When the basal ganglia are disrupted by the brain inflammation, serious changes in behavior and thought processes can occur. [498]

---

[496] Barkley, R.A. (1997) *ADHD and the nature of self-control.* New York: Guilford Press.

[497] de Oliveira, S.K. & Pelajo, C.F. (March 2010) Pediatric Autoimmune Neuropsychiatric Disorders Associated with Streptococcal Infection (PANDAS): a Controversial Diagnosis. *Curr Infect Dis Rep* 12 (2): 103–9. doi:10.1007/s11908-010-0082-7

[498] Pichichero, M.E. (2009) The PANDAS syndrome. *Adv Exp Med Biol. Advances in Experimental Medicine and Biology* (Springer) 634: 205–16. doi:10.1007/978-0-387-79838-7_17

The original PANDAS diagnostic criteria specified that the associated symptoms were hyperactivity (ADHD) or other motor symptoms, but experience has shown that the list is longer. A combination of neuropsychiatric symptoms can occur, such as

- OCD + tics + ADHD-like symptoms;
- OCD + severe separation anxiety + bedwetting;
- OCD + tics + hyperactivity + developmental regression.

The possible combinations are too numerous to list, but in all cases, the associated symptoms should begin at the same time as the OCD (or within 1 – 2 days) and have an equally dramatic, sudden onset. The most common accompanying symptoms are:

- Severe separation anxiety (e.g., child can't leave parent's side or needs to sleep on floor next to parent's bed, etc.)
- Generalized anxiety. which may progress to episodes of panic and a "terror-stricken look"
- Motoric hyperactivity, abnormal movements, and a sense of restlessness
- Sensory abnormalities, including hyper-sensitivity to light or sounds, distortions of visual perceptions, and occasionally, visual or auditory hallucinations
- Concentration difficulties, and loss of academic abilities, particularly in math and visual-spatial areas
- Increased urinary frequency and a new onset of bed-wetting
- Irritability (sometimes with aggression) and emotional changes. Abrupt onset of depression can also occur, with thoughts about suicide.

- Developmental regression, including temper tantrums, "baby talk" and handwriting deterioration (also related to motor symptoms)
- Sleep disturbance [499]

To diagnose a current or recent Streptococcal infection the following tests are available:

- A throat swab (rapid Strep test or throat swab culture) can identify a current case of Strep throat
- An ASO titre (antistrepolysin titre) shows an elevation in antibodies to Strep 3-6 weeks after infection
- An AntiDNAase-B titre (antistreptococcal DNAase B titre) shows an elevation in antibodies to Strep 6-8 weeks after infection [500]

A positive result in any of these tests does not diagnose PANDAS, it just gives more information about whether the child has had a recent exposure to Strep. In addition, low Strep titres do not rule out PANDAS. If symptoms of PANDAS occur suddenly, it is useful to have the above Strep titres tested to see if a recent Strep infection could be related.

Beyond this point, further testing for food allergies or sensitivities, as well as levels of immunoglobulins (IgE,

---

[499] de Oliveira, S.K. & Pelajo, C.F. (March 2010) Pediatric Autoimmune Neuropsychiatric Disorders Associated with Streptococcal Infection (PANDAS): a Controversial Diagnosis. *Curr Infect Dis Rep* 12 (2): 103–9. doi:10.1007/s11908-010-0082-7

[500] Swedo, S.E., Leckman, J.F. & Rose, N.R. (2012) From research subgroup to clinical syndrome: Modifying the PANDAS criteria to describe PANS (Pediatric Acute-onset Neuropsychiatric Syndrome). *Pediatr Therapeut* 2012, 2:2.

IgG, IgA, and IgM) can be done to assess for additional burden on the immune system that is contributing to the susceptibility to PANDAS. [501]

*TREATMENT*

Treatment for PANDAS may include oral antibiotics to eradicate a Streptococcal infection, and prophylactic antibiotics to prevent recurrence. Oral prednisone is also used as a potent anti-inflammatory to relieve inflammation of the brain and prevent damage. Another therapy known as intravenous immunoglobulin (IVIG) is being investigated.[502]

Complementary treatments support the use of antibiotics with probiotics (non-Streptococcal strains), and natural therapies to down regulate inflammation and support the brain, such as curcumin, EPA and DHA. Vitamins and minerals to support immune function (vitamin C, B vitamins, zinc, and selenium) should be administered intravenously. Intravenous glutathione, a potent antioxidant, can be used to protect the brain from being damaged from inflammation. [503]

Investigation should be done to rule out or treat other non-Streptococcal infections that may be present such as Candida (yeast), parasites, viruses (EBV, CMV, HSV),

---

[501] Murphy, T.K., Storch, E.A., Lewin, A.B., Edge, P.J. & Goodman, W.K. (2012) Clinical factors associated with pediatric autoimmune neuropsychiatric disorders associated with streptococcal infections. *J Pediatr. 2012 Feb;160(2):314-9.*

[502] Snider LA, Swedo SE. PANDAS: current status and directions for research. *Mol Psychiatry.* 2004 Oct;9(10):900-

[503] Murphy, M.L. & Pichichero, M.E. (2002) Prospective identification and treatment of children with pediatric autoimmune neuropsychiatric disorder associated with group A streptococcal infection (PANDAS). *Arch Pediatr Adolesc Med.* 2002 Apr;156(4):356-61.

Lyme disease, or pathogenic bacterial overgrowth.[446] Food allergy and food sensitivity testing can be done, and foods should be eliminated from the diet that may be placing additional burden on the immune system.

Although all these treatments can be very effective, a change in lifestyle might also be important. Children with recurrent Strep infections may be constantly re-infected with the Strep bacteria through a family member that carries the bacteria without symptoms. A child may also be re-exposed to Strep through skin infection (impetigo), urinary tract infection or ear infection. Immune system support to prevent recurrence of these conditions is important in long-term management of PANDAS. The tonsils and adenoids may hide Streptococcal bacteria and some evidence suggests tonsil and adenoid removal in cases of PANDAS; however, careful consideration of the role of the tonsils and adenoids in fighting infection should be made before making this decision.[504]

## ADHD AND SLEEP DISORDERS

Not every child with ADHD has sleep issues, but it can happen. In one study, about half the parents said their child with ADHD had difficulty sleeping. Parents reported that their child felt tired when they woke up, had nightmares, or had other sleep problems such as sleep apnea or restless legs syndrome. Another study

---

[504] Murphy, T.K., Storch, E.A., Lewin, A.B., Edge, P.J. & Goodman, W.K. (2012) Clinical factors associated with pediatric autoimmune neuropsychiatric disorders associated with streptococcal infections. *J Pediatr. 2012 Feb;160(2):314-9.*

involving children with ADHD found the children had less refreshing sleep, difficulty getting up, and more daytime sleepiness. [505]

## IS SNORING RELATED TO *ADHD?*

Large tonsils and adenoids can partially block the airway at night. This can cause snoring and poor sleep. That, in turn, may lead to attention problems the next day. In one study of 5- to 7-year-olds, snoring was more common among children with mild ADHD than in the other children. In another study, kids who snored were almost twice as likely as their peers to have ADHD. However, that doesn't prove that snoring caused ADHD.
Children who snore tend to score worse on tests of attention, language abilities, and overall intelligence. These children may have sleep apnea. [506]

## SLEEP APNEA

People with sleep apnea have brief episodes when they stop breathing, though they don't know it. These episodes can happen frequently throughout the night. Enlarged tonsils and adenoids are the most common causes of sleep apnea in children. But obesity and chronic allergies can also be a cause.

---

[505] Mairav Cohen-Zion, Sonia Ancoli-Israelb, (2004) Sleep In Children With Attention-Deficit Hyperactivity Disorder (ADHD): A Review Of Naturalistic And Stimulant Intervention Studies. *Sleep Med Reviews,* Volume 8, Issue 5, October 2004, Pages 379–402

[506] Cohen-Zion,M. & Ancoli-Israel, S. (2004)Sleep in children with attention-deficit hyperactivity disorder (ADHD): a review of naturalistic and stimulant intervention studies. *Sleep Medicine Reviews,* Volume 8, Issue 5, October 2004, Pages 379–402

As with adults, children with sleep apnea are tired during the day. They may have problems concentrating and might have other symptoms related to lack of sleep such as irritability.

Sleep apnea in children is treatable. Your pediatrician or an ear, nose, and throat specialist can determine whether your child's tonsils are enlarged enough to possibly block the airway and cause sleep apnea.[507]

To confirm the diagnosis, the child may complete a sleep study that's done in a special laboratory. Not every child with enlarged tonsils or with loud snoring has sleep apnea.

Surgery is the treatment of choice for kids with enlarged tonsils and adenoids. Other treatments are available for those with restricted nighttime breathing due to allergies or other causes.

## Neurotherapy and ADHD

The inability to maintain focus and control impulsivity is typical with those who have ADHD. Using HEG neurofeedback reveals these failures of attention on the computer screen as they are happening. Wandering thoughts and lack of focus is obvious. To change this behavior we know that brain plasticity will change how our brain functions just by repetition. Ultimately, these changes become habits requiring no conscious effort.

---

[507] Friedman, M, Samuelson, C. G., Hamilton, C, Maley, A, Taylor, D. Kelley, K. eta al (2012) Modified Adenotonsillectomy to Improve Cure Rates for Pediatric Obstructive Sleep Apnea: A Randomized Controlled Trial. Otolaryngol Head Neck Surg July 2012 vol. 147 no. 1 132-138

Classical EEG neurofeedback meets the ADHD challenge by repeated sessions devoted to training the electrical activity of the brain. HEG, on the other hand, trains to improve blood flow and oxygenation in the brain where focus is constantly measured. This measurement is continuously displayed so the client can maximize their results. At the end of each session attention is recorded, graphed, and presented for progress evaluation.

Clinical trials show this technique is very effective at allowing the individual control over their results, giving them a tool to use outside the clinic. It helps them to calm down anxiety, impulsivity and focus issues while allowing them to slow down and think more clearly. We have also found it helps rid them of sensory integration issues which make extraneous sounds and lights so distracting.

Neurotherapy has also been found to be very cost-effective. A review of published literature identified 13 studies, most conducted on existing databases by using diagnostic and medical procedure codes and focused on health care costs. Costs were examined for ADHD treatment-related and other health care costs, special education, disciplinary costs, and parental work loss.

Based on this small evidence base, the estimated annual COI of ADHD in children and adolescents was $14,576 per individual (2005 dollars). Given the variability of estimates across studies on which that number is based, a reasonable range is between

$12,005 and $17,458 per individual.[508] On the contrary, neurotherapy can make a permanent change in just a few weeks. Many insurance providers are now covering neurotherapy, and their reimbursement rates are comparable to other treatments.

## CONCLUSION

We live in a busy society. Cellphones, email and even Twitter limited to 140 characters can interrupt concentration. Contrary to the belief that multitasking is what it takes to get ahead in business or the world, our brains don't multitask. As evidenced by the so-called "attentional-blink" deficit, the information processing capacity of the human mind is limited. In this example, when two targets blink rapidly on and off, frequently the second target is not seen. This deficit is believed to result from competition between the two targets for limited attentional resources. The good news is that attention can be learned. Although many parents are swayed by the idea that a pill will be the answer to all their children's attention and focus issues, alternative treatments such as neurotherapy, nutrition counseling and elimination of toxins and heavy metals in the system is a better and more permanent path.

According to the April, 2009 study by Elizabeth Zelinski, Ph.D., older adults as well as children can improve memory and attention by training on

---

[508] Pelham, W., Foster, E. & Robb, J. (2009) The Economic Impact of Attention-Deficit/Hyperactivity Disorder in Children and Adolescents Ambulatory Pediatrics, 7(1), 121-131.

computerized brain exercises.[509] Dr. Zelinski, at the annual meeting of the American Geriatrics Society in Chicago reported on new data showing that the gains persist months after the training ended.

Dr. Zelinski's study was referred to as *"An IMPACT Study: A randomized controlled trial of a brain plasticity-based training program for age-related decline"*. This study had a total of 487 healthy adults over the age of 65 participate. Half were assigned to a group that trained on a brain fitness software program for 40 hours over eight weeks. The other half spent an equal amount of time attending to lectures via computer and answering quizzes.

The study found that participants who trained with cognitive software, more than doubled their processing speed, with an average increase of 131%. They also saw gains on standard measures of memory and attention of 10 years, on average. These changes were big enough that participants reported significant improvements in everyday activities (such as remembering names or understanding conversations in noisy restaurants). The gains of the brain exercise group were clinically significant; the gains of the lecture group were significantly smaller and not clinically significant.

---

[509] Smith, G. E., Housen, P., Yaffe, K., Ruff, R., Kennison, R. F., Mahncke, H. W., & Zelinski, E. M. (2009). A Cognitive Training Program Based on Principles of Brain Plasticity: Results from the Improvement in Memory with Plasticity-based Adaptive Cognitive Training (IMPACT) Study. *Journal of the American Geriatrics Society, 57*(4), 594-603.

So for those who have ADHD there is an answer. Neurotherapy offers an alternative to dangerous drugs and years of failure. It is an easy way to retrain your brain to function optimally for better attention and focus and to lessen impulsivity.

# CHAPTER 13
# MEMORY LOSS

Our memory gives us the ability to retain and recall incidents and information. But more importantly, it allows us a sense of self, to feel comfortable with those we know and to use past experiences as a guide in new situations. However, our memory doesn't always work perfectly.

It can be affected by brain injury, stress, diet, and lack of sleep, medications, lack of exercise, alcohol and drug abuse as well as natural aging. As people grow older, it may take longer to retrieve memories. Some adults joke about having a "senior moment." However, sometimes memory loss can be more serious or even life-threatening.

## WHAT IS MEMORY?

Memory isn't a thing you can see or hold in your hand. It doesn't even happen in a single part of our brain. Memory is a brain-wide process.[510] Each memory can have several components. If you are remembering a painting, you could have memories of the colors, the smell of the paint and the feel of the surface.

---

[510] Salmon, E., Van der Linden, M., Collette, F., Delfiore, G., Maquet, P., Degueldre, C. et al. (2005) Neurophysiological architecture of functional magnetic resonance images of human brain. Cereb Cortex , 15, 1332-42.

Each sensation is stored in a different area of the brain. The entire image of "the painting" is actively reconstructed by the brain from all those different areas. Neurologists are only beginning to understand how the parts are reassembled into a coherent whole.

## MEMORY ENCODING

The first step in creating a memory is encoding. It's a biological phenomenon that begins with perception. The combination of different sensory information received. For example, think of your first car.

When you first saw it your visual cortex registered physical features such as the shape and the color. Your auditory system registered the sound as the engine ran and the squeak of the door as it opened. The olfactory system registered the smell of the leather seats. The feel of the smooth metal is also recorded in your memory. The hippocampus receives information about each of these memories. It integrates these perceptions and provides a single multifaceted memory of that one occasion.

For these memories to be stored in your long-term memory, the hippocampus and the frontal cortex analyze these sensory inputs and decide if they're worth remembering. The storage of these memories uses electrochemical communication. Neurons connect with other neighboring neurons through synapses when you experience something new.

As more and more cells are added, a neural network is formed. The more signals being sent between these neurons, the stronger the network becomes. With each new experience, your brain is slightly rewired by adding connections. The more information you gain, the more connections are made reinforcing the network. However, these connections can also be pruned away when you stop using the information. When this happens you start to forget what you once knew.[511]

## MEMORY RETRIEVAL

The memories stored must be retrieved in order to be used. In other words, new memories start life as a temporary excitation of synapses in a network of neurons. If you recall a memory, the same neural pathways are reactivated. The more times these pathways are reactivated, the stronger the memory becomes and the more likely it is to be converted into a long-term memory. There are four basic ways in which the information can be pulled from long-term memory. The retrieval cues, or prompts that are available to trigger the recovery of long-term memory, can have an impact on how the information is reclaimed.[512]

- Recall: This type of memory retrieval involves access to events or information from the past without being reminded of any part of the memory. Remembering a vacation or being able to answer questions on a fill-in-the-blank test is a good example of recall.

[511] Foster, J.K. (2002) The Oxford Handbook of Memory. Brain, 125 (2), 439-441.
[512] Stern, P., Chin, G. & Travis, J. (2004) Neuroscience: Higher Brain Functions. Science, 306 (5695), 431. doi: 10.1126/science.306.5695.431

- Recollection: This type of memory retrieval involves reconstructing memory, from fragments or partial memories of the information or event. For example, writing an answer on an essay exam often starts with remembering small bits of information, and then those memories trigger more information based on these initial memories.
- Recognition: This type of memory retrieval involves correctly remembering information that has been experienced before. For example, taking a multiple choice quiz requires you to recognize the correct answer out of a group of available answers.
- Relearning: This type of memory retrieval involves relearning information that has been previously learned. Relearning often makes the memory stronger and therefore easier to remember and retrieve in the future.

## PROBLEMS WITH RETRIEVAL

Unfortunately, the retrieval process is not always accurate. Knowing you know the answer but not being able to dredge it up out of your memory is called a "tip of the tongue" experience. While you may know this information is stored somewhere in your memory, you are unable to access and retrieve it. Sometimes you may even be able to remember the first letter of the word you're seeking.[513]

Although this can be troubling to most of us, for someone worried about possible dementia, it can be devastating. The good news is that research has shown

---

[513] Brown, A.S. (1991) A review of the tip-of-the-tongue experience. *Psychological Bulletin, 109* (2), 204-223.

that these experiences are  extremely common, typically occurring at least once each week for most younger individuals, and two to four times per week for elderly adults.[514]

## Types of Memory

There are three main components of memory. They are sense memory, short-term memory (also known as working memory) and long-term memory.

### *Sense Memory*

Sense memory involves the connection between memory and the senses and how sensory stimuli can trigger memories. Researchers who work with memory have learned that the five senses (sight, hearing, touch, smell and taste) can play a very significant role in the process of making, storing, and retrieving memories.[515] Smell for example can be very evocative. As the olfactory bulb is located next to that part of the brain that handles memory storage, people tend to create strong links between smells and particular memories.

Many of us have strong associations with a variety of smells, ranging from "my lover's perfume" to "one really good meal." Smell is used in marketing to trigger those past memories to encourage people to buy. The smell of popcorn in a movie theater or the smell of

---

[514] Schacter, D.L. (2001) The seven sins of memory: How the mind forgets and remembers. New York: Houghton Mifflin.
[515] Wesson, D. W. & Wilson, D. A. (2010) Smelling Sounds: Olfactory-auditory convergence in the olfactory tubercle. *J Neurosci.* *30*(3013),1021. PMID 20181598.

freshly baked cookies in an open house for sale is good examples of smell-induced memories for marketing.[516]

## Short-term Memory

Short-term memory is also known as working memory. It stores information that you need only remember for seconds, minutes or hours. An example would be a grocery list given to you verbally that you must remember until you get to the grocery store. Short-term memory is believed to rely mostly on an auditory code for storing information, and to a lesser extent visual code. This type of memory is supported by regions of the frontal lobe (especially dorsolateral prefrontal cortex) and the parietal lobe.[517]

## Long-term Memory

Long-term memory has a much larger capacity and these memories are harder to forget. Long-term memory retains those important memories such as names of family and friends, your address, as well as information on how and when to do certain activities and tasks. Long-term memories are stored by more stable and permanent changes in neural connections widely spread throughout the brain.

There are actually two kinds of long-term memory, explicit memory (learned memory) and implicit

---

[516] Lundström, J. N., Boyle, J. A,, Zatorre, R. J., & Jones-Gotman, M. (2009) The neuronal substrates of human olfactory based kin recognition. *Hum Brain Mapp. 30*, 2571–2580. PMID 19067327

[517] Conrad, R. (1964) Acoustic Confusions in Immediate Memory. *British Journal of Psychology, 55*, 75-84.

memory for unconscious, non-intentional form of memory.[518]

## Explicit Memory

Explicit memory is the conscious, intentional recollection of previous experiences and information. We constantly use explicit memory throughout the day, such as remembering that doctor's appointment or recalling an event from years ago. A good example of explicit memory is remembering when you learned to draw or ride a bike.

Explicit memory involves several neural structures. Most are in the temporal lobe or closely related, such as the amygdala, the hippocampus, the rhinal cortex in the temporal lobe, and the prefrontal cortex. There are two types of explicit memory, episodic and semantic.[519]

### Episodic Memory

Episodic memory is associated with the hippocampus which also regulates the body's stress response. Lynn Nadel, Ph.D., from Arizona State University and his colleagues found that stress increased false-memory rates.[520] According to Nadel, "They asked participants to give a 10-minute speech to a panel of judges. Then,

---

[518] Salmon, E., Van der Linden, M., Collette, F., Delfiore, G., Maquet, P., Degueldre, C. et al. (2005) Neurophysiological architecture of functional magnetic resonance images of human brain. *Cereb Cortex*, *15*, 1332-42.

[519] Foster, J.K. (2002) *The Oxford Handbook of Memory. Brain*, *125* (2), 439-441.

[520] Nadel, L. & Payne, J. D. (2002) The relationship between episodic memory and context: Clues from memory errors made while under stress. Physiol. Res., Suppl 1( 51), S3–S11.

---

those stressed participants and some unstressed control participants listened to a long word list. Later, the stressed participants were more likely to say that they remembered hearing words that were not really on the list."

*Semantic Memory*

Semantic memory consists of all explicit memory that is not autobiographical. Examples of semantic memory are knowledge of historical events and figures, the ability to recognize friends and acquaintances, and information learned in school, such as specialized vocabularies and reading, writing and mathematics.

The neural basis of episodic and semantic memory is not yet known. However, some scientists suggest that episodic memory may be dependent upon the right side of the brain, while semantic memory dependent on the left.[521]

# Implicit Memory

Implicit Memory includes those things you remember without being aware that you are remembering them such as brushing your teeth in the morning. It is an automatic or an unconscious form of memory. [522,523] Although there are large age-related differences with

---

[521] Tulving, E. & Schacter, D. L. (1990) Priming and human memory systems. *Science, 247* (4940), 301 – 306. doi: 10.1126/science.2296719

[522] Schaechter, J.D., Wurtman ,R.J. (1990) Serotonin release varies with brain tryptophan levels. *Brain Res. 532*(1-2), 203–10. doi:10.1016/0006-8993(90)91761-5.

[523] Benjamin, L. T. ,Hopkins, J. R., & Nation, J. R. (1994) *Psychology (3rd edition)*. New York: Macmillan College Publishing Company.

explicit memory, age has little or no effect on implicit memory.

Implicit memory is unique as most amnesiacs and those suffering from memory loss and dementia still have implicit memory skills even if they don't realize it. This helps explain why elderly people are often more comfortable and capable when they stay in a familiar place. Years of living in the same rooms with the same furnishings produces implicit memories such as knowing where to find a broom and other useful information. When an elderly person is put in a nursing home or other unfamiliar environment, the same person may seem disabled, because none of the old automatic routines work in the new environment.[524] There are two basic types of implicit memory; *Priming* and *Procedural Memory*.

## *Priming*

Priming occurs when previous information facilitates later processing of that information. You are "primed" by your experiences; if you have heard something very recently, or many more times than another thing, you are primed to recall it more quickly. This phenomenon has been seen in studies when subjects are exposed to a set of words and then later tested. Later tests consist of priming subjects with parts of a word and asking them to complete the word with whatever comes to mind. The results of these tests are that subjects are

---

[524] Cohen, N.J., Eichenbaum, H., Deacedo, B.S., & Corkin, S. (1985) Different memory systems underlying acquisition of procedural and declarative knowledge. *Annals of the New York Academy of Sciences, 444*, 54-71.

likely to complete the word to match words they were exposed to at the beginning. This type of learning is one type of implicit memory.

## Procedural Memory

Procedural memory consists of learned, automatic movements or skills. These memories are only accessed by using or executing them. It's our "how to" knowledge. Riding a bike, tying a shoe and washing dishes are all tasks that require procedural memory. Even what we think of as "natural" tasks, such as walking, require procedural memory.[525] Though we can do such tasks fairly easily, it's often hard to verbalize exactly how we do them. Procedural memory likely uses a different part of the brain than episodic memory. That's why a person who has experienced amnesia and forgets much about his or her personal life often retains procedural memory: how to use a fork or throw a baseball, for example.

In a 2007 study, Jessica D. Payne and her colleagues showed a series of slides that told a story—either an emotional story or a neutral one—to participants. When the researchers asked the participants to recall the story one week later, they found that stressing the participant before the emotional story actually increased memory, but stressing the participant before the neutral story decreased memory.[526]

---

[525] Squire, L. R. (2004) Memory systems of the brain: A brief history and current perspective. Neurobiology of Learning and Memory. *82*,171-177.

[526] Nadel, L. & Payne, J. D. (2002) The relationship between episodic memory and context: Clues from memory errors made while under stress. *Physiol. Res., Suppl 1(* 51), S3–S11.

According to Nadel, research shows that "...aversive events that happen early in life can leave powerful traces behind, but with no record of where or when these experiences occurred." He concluded that this could explain strong phobias that have no known cause, or even post-traumatic stress disorder.

## Brain Anatomy Related to Memory

Memory is stored in several areas of the brain. However, we can see the primary structures and the memory types that relate to it from studying damaged brains in the past. The following is a short overview of structures in the brain and memory functions that relate to them.[527]

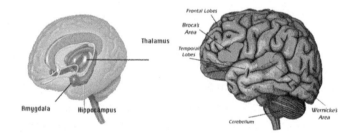

**Fig. 13-1 Areas of Memory function**

The **Cerebellum** is where procedural memories are maintained.

The **Hippocampus** is involved in transferring memories from short term to long term memory. Some of this process is thought to occur during sleep.[528] The

---

[527] Kolb, B. & Whishaw, I. (2003) *Fundamentals of Human Neuropsychology*. New York: Worth Publishers.

[528] Benjamin, L. T. ,Hopkins, J. R., & Nation, J. R. (1994) *Psychology (3rd edition)*. New York: Macmillan College Publishing Company.

hippocampus is also thought to be involved in spatial memories, such as recognizing a road route.[529]

The **Thalamus** is thought, in combination with the hippocampus, to be involved in spatial memories. It is also thought to be involved in emotional memories. It also may be involved in actually forming the original memory before encoding takes place.

The **Amygdala** is in charge of strong emotions. Because of this, it is also closely tied to memory. The degree and type of emotional impact of an event has a great influence on an event being stored in memory. If a person experiences something extremely emotional, the amygdala will activate connections with the hippocampus so that the event will be more memorable.[530]

The **Temporal Lobes** are very important in the storage of past events. [256] Also, Wernicke's area, located in the temporal lobe is an area related to understanding language. Broca's Area is related to speech and is located in the frontal lobes. Damage to this area in the brain can result in aphasia. [256]

## MEMORIZATION

There are many ways humans use tools to remember an object or thing. Memorization methods have been

[529] Cardoso, S. H. (2000) *Loss of Memory*. State University of Campinas. Center for Biomedical Informatics. Retrieved from: http://www.epub.org/Br/cm/n01/memo/loss_i.htm

[530] Cardoso, S. H. (1997) How to Improve Your Memory. *State University of Campinas. Center for Biomedical Informatics.* Retrieved from: http://www.epub.org/Br/cm/n01/memo/improve_i.htm

the subject of much discussion over the years. In 1579, Cosmos Rossellius, a Florentine Dominican friar wrote a book describing "visual alphabets." He showed that a spacing effect shows that an individual is more likely to remember a list of items when rehearsal is spaced over an extended period of time. Intense memorization, or cramming, is a way to remember something in a short period of time. Also the "Zeigarnik effect" states that people remember uncompleted or interrupted tasks better than completed ones.[531]

Odors used to reactivate memories were used by German researchers in 2007. The researchers found they could use odors to re-activate new memories in individuals while they slept and they remembered better later.[532] Interference or inhibition can also hinder memorization and retrieval. This theorizes that forgetting at the behavioral level is anchored in the phenomenon of interference, or inhibition, which can be either retroactive or proactive.

- Retroactive inhibition is where new learning interferes with the retention of old memories.
- Proactive inhibition is where old memories interfere with the retention of new learning.

Emotion can have a powerful impact on memory. Numerous studies have shown that the most vivid autobiographical memories tend to be of emotional

---

[531] Baumeister, R. F., & Bushman, B. J. (2008) *Social Psychology and Human Nature*. United States: Thompson Wadsworth.
[532] Reuters (2007) Smell of Roses May Improve Memory. March 12, 2007. Retrieved from:
http://archive.newsmax.com/archives/articles/2007/3/12/90015.shtm

events, which are likely to be recalled more often and with more clarity and detail than neutral events.[533]

## Stress and Memory

During periods of stress, our bodies secrete a stress hormone called cortisol which can interfere with the energy supply to certain brain cells involved in memory. Too much cortisol can prevent the brain from laying down a new memory or from accessing already existing memories.

Robert M. Sapolsky, Ph.D., professor of Biological Sciences, Neurology and Neurological Sciences at Stanford, demonstrated that sustained stress can damage the hippocampus, the part of the limbic brain which is central to learning and memory. The culprits are "glucocorticoids," a class of steroid hormones secreted from the adrenal glands during stress. They are more commonly known as corticosteroids or cortisol.[534]

During a perceived threat, the adrenal glands immediately release adrenalin.[535] If the threat is severe or still persists after a couple of minutes, the adrenals then release cortisol. Once in the brain, cortisol

---

[533] Christianson, S.A.,& Loftus, E. (1990) Some characteristics of people's traumatic memories. *Bulletin of the Psychonomic Society, 28,* 195-198.

[534] Sapolsky, R.M (1992) Stress, the Aging Brain, and the Mechanisms of Neuron Death. Cambridge: MIT Press.

[535] Sternberg, E. (2001) The Balance Within: The Science Connecting Health and Emotions.Plymouth, MI: W. H. Freeman and Company

remains for a much longer period than adrenalin, where it continues to affect brain cells.[536]

Have you ever forgotten something during a stressful situation that you should have remembered? Cortisol also interferes with the function of neurotransmitters, the chemicals that brain cells use to communicate with each other.

Excessive cortisol can make it difficult to think or retrieve long-term memories. That's why people get befuddled and confused in a severe crisis. Their mind goes blank because "the lines are down." For example, they can't remember where the fire exit is. [260]

Blood glucose is diverted by stress hormones to exercise muscles; therefore, the amount of glucose (or energy) that reaches the brain's hippocampus is diminished. This creates an energy crisis in the hippocampus which compromises its ability to create new memories.[537] This may be the reason some people can't remember a very traumatic event, and why short-term memory is usually the first casualty of age-related memory loss resulting from a lifetime of stress.

In a 1998 study at the University of California at Irvine, an elevated level of a stress hormone hindered the ability of rats to find their way back to a hidden target. Rats were stressed by an electrical shock and then sent through a maze with which they were already familiar. When the shock was given either four hours before or

---

[536] Gleitman, H.,. Fridlund, A.J. & Reisberg, D. (2004) *Psychology, 6*, NY: Norton.
[537] Friedman, H. S., & Silver, R. C. (Eds). (2007) *Foundations of Health Psychology*. New York: Oxford University Press

two minutes before navigating the maze, the rats had no problem. But, when they were stressed by a shock 30 minutes before, the rats were unable to remember their way through the maze.[538]

This time-dependent effect on memory performance correlates with the levels of circulating cortisol, which are highest at 30 minutes after a stressing event. The same thing occurred when non-stressed rats were injected with cortisol. In contrast, when cortisol production was chemically suppressed, then there were no stress-induced effects on memory retrieval.[539]

According to James McGaugh, director of the Center for the Neurobiology of Learning and Memory at the University of California, Irvine, "This effect only lasts for a couple of hours, so that the impairing effect in this case is a temporary impairment of retrieval. The memory is not lost. It is just inaccessible or less accessible for a period of time." [540]

Normally, in response to stress, the brain's hypothalamus secretes a hormone that causes the pituitary gland to secrete another hormone that causes the adrenals to secrete cortisol. When levels of cortisol

---

[538] Roozendaal, B., de Quervain, D.J., Ferry, B., Setlow, B., & McGaugh, J. L. ( 2001) Basolateral amygdala-nucleus accumbens interactions in mediating glucocorticoid enhancement of memory consolidation. *J. Neurosci. 21*,2518–2525.

[539] Lupien, S.J., Wilkinson, C.J., Brière, S., Ng Ying Kin, N.M.K., Meaney, M.J. & Nair, P.V. (2002) Acute Modulation of Aged Human Memory by Pharmacological Manipulation of Glucocorticoids. *The Journal of Clinical Endocrinology & Metabolism, 87* (8), 3798-3807.

[540] deQuervain, D. J., Roozendaal, B. & McGaugh, J. L. (1998) Stress and glucocorticoids impair retrieval of long-term spatial memory , *Nature* 394:787-90

rise to a certain level, several areas of the brain—especially the hippocampus—tell the hypothalamus to turn off the cortisol-producing mechanism; this is the proper feedback response.[541]

The hippocampus, however, is the area most damaged by cortisol. In his book Brain Longevity, Dharma Singh Khalsa, M.D., describes the effect of loss of hippocampal cells on the control of cortisol secretion. When older people have lost 20-25% of the cells in their hippocampus, it is unable to provide proper feedback to the hypothalamus and cortisol continues to be secreted. This, in turn, causes more damage to the hippocampus, and even more cortisol production. Thus, a Catch-22 "degenerative cascade" begins, which can be very difficult to stop.[542]

## ALZHEIMER'S DISEASE

Just like the rest of our bodies, our brains change as we age. Most of us notice some slowed thinking and occasional problems with remembering certain things. However, serious memory loss, confusion and other major changes in the way our minds work are not a normal part of aging. They may be a sign that brain cells are failing. Alzheimer's disease (AD) is a brain disorder named for German physician Alois Alzheimer, who first described it in 1906.

---

[541] Engelmann, M., Landgraf ,R. & Wotjak, C. (2004) The hypothalamic-neurohypophysial system regulates the hypothalamic-pituitary-adrenal axis under stress: an old concept revisited. Front Neuroendocrinol 25 (3-4), 132–49. oi:10.1016/j.yfrne.2004.09.001. PMID 15589266

[542] Khalsa, D. S. (1999) Brain Longevity: The Breakthrough Medical Program that Improves Your Mind and Memory. Boston: Grand Central Publishing.

In the past century, scientists have learned a great deal about Alzheimer's disease. The most important is that AD is not inevitable. There are actions you can take to increase your resistance and stave off AD's effects.[543]

Within the human brain there is a complex mix of chemical and electrical processes. Alzheimer's disease disrupts this intricate signaling system. This disruption occurs from the creation of two abnormal structures in the brain called amyloid plaques and neurofibrillary tangles. Plaques are composed of beta amyloid, a toxic molecule that originates in normal protein. Something causes enzymes in the brain to cut this protein into fragments that then clump together into damaging plaques. Normally, tau proteins stabilize the internal support structure of neurons, but in Alzheimer's disease, the tau protein threads become entangled, killing the neuron by damaging critical parts of its transport system. As the disease progresses, more neurons die, the brain shrinks, and memory is lost.[544]

According to the 2009 *Alzheimer's Disease Facts and Figures*, published by the Alzheimer's Association:

1.  Memory changes that disrupt daily life. One of the most common signs of AD, especially in its early stages, is forgetting recently learned information. Others include forgetting important dates or

---

[543] Waldemar G, Dubois B, Emre M, et al. (January 2007) Recommendations for the diagnosis and management of Alzheimer's disease and other disorders associated with dementia: EFNS guideline. *Eur J Neurol* 14(1), e1–26.

[544] Tiraboschi, P, Hansen, LA, Thal, LJ, & Corey-Bloom, J. (2004) The importance of neuritic plaques and tangles to the development and evolution of AD. *Neurology, 62* (11), 1984–9. PMID 15184601

events; asking for the same information over and over, relying on memory aides (e.g., reminder notes or electronic devices) or family members for things they used to handle on their own.

2.  Challenges in planning or solving problems. Some people may experience changes in their ability to develop and follow a plan or work with numbers. They may have trouble following a familiar recipe or keeping track of monthly bills. They may have difficulty concentrating and take much longer to do things than they did before.

3.  Difficulty completing familiar tasks at home, at work or at leisure. People with AD often find it hard to complete daily tasks. Sometimes, people may have trouble driving to a familiar location, managing a budget at work or remembering the rules of a favorite game.

4.  Confusion with time or place. People with AD can lose track of dates, seasons and the passage of time. They may have trouble understanding something if it is not happening immediately. Sometimes they may forget where they are or how they got there.

5.  Trouble understanding visual images and spatial relationships. For some people, vision problems are a sign of AD. They may have difficulty reading, judging distance and determining color or contrast. In terms of perception, they may pass a mirror and think someone else is in the room. They may not realize they are the person in the mirror.

6.  New problems with words in speaking or writing. People with AD may have trouble following or joining a conversation. They may stop in the middle of a conversation and have no idea how to continue or they may repeat themselves. They may struggle

with vocabulary, have problems finding the right word or call things by the wrong name (e.g., calling a "watch" a "hand-clock").

7. Misplacing things and losing the ability to retrace steps. A person with AD may put things in unusual places. They may lose things and be unable to go back over their steps to find them again. Sometimes, they may accuse others of stealing. This may occur more frequently over time.

8. Decreased or poor judgment. People with AD may experience changes in judgment or decision-making. For example, they may use poor judgment when dealing with money, giving large amounts to telemarketers. They may pay less attention to grooming or keeping themselves clean.

9. Withdrawal from work or social activities. A person with AD may start to remove themselves from hobbies, social activities, work projects or sports. They may have trouble keeping up with a favorite sports team or remembering how to complete a favorite hobby. They may also avoid being social because of the changes they have experienced.

10. Changes in mood and personality. The mood and personalities of people with AD can change. They can become confused, suspicious, depressed, fearful or anxious. They may be easily upset at home, at work, with friends or in places where they are out of their comfort zone.

In 1986, Dr. David Snowdon, then at the University of Minnesota, began a scientific study involving 678 Catholic nuns from the School Sisters of Notre Dame. This research project, often called the "Nun Study," is one of the most significant long-term research studies ever done on aging and Alzheimer's disease.[545]

One of the primary questions the Nun Study researchers attempted to answer was how pathology in the human brain related to AD symptoms. Over the period of the study, the only method to determine brain pathology was through autopsy on deceased study participants.

During autopsy, researchers observed physical changes in the brains of the study participants. They then attempted to relate their pathological observations back to the lifetime behavior observed in the participant.

One of their research questions was: Did every participant with AD-related physical brain changes display symptoms of AD while alive? The results from the Nun Study were exciting. They showed that approximately one-third of the sisters whose brains had displayed post-mortem AD changes (plaques and tangles) had shown no behavioral symptoms of dementia while alive. In fact, these women scored normal results in all mental and physical tests! The researchers hypothesized that the reason they were unaffected was Cognitive Reserve.

Cognition is defined as the process of thought and includes communication, problem-solving, learning and memory. Cognitive Reserve lets individuals with greater cognitive skills delay symptoms of AD in spite

---

[545] Snowdon D. (2003) Healthy aging and dementia: Findings from the Nun Study. *Annals of Internal Medicine* 139 (5 Part 2):450454, 2003.

of underlying changes occurring in their brains. Lifestyles including intellectual pursuits, physical activities, and socializing are associated with slower cognitive decline in the healthy older set.

There is also evidence from functional imaging studies that subjects engaging in such activities can clinically tolerate more AD pathology. It is possible that training your brain and body creates more efficient cognitive function and therefore delays the onset of dementia.[546]

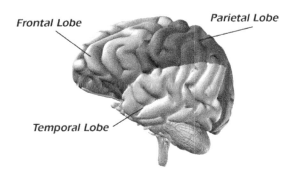

©Andreas Meyer - Fotolia.com

**Fig. 13-2 Areas of the brain affected by Alzheimer's Disease**

Figure 13-2 shows the left side view of the brain including areas commonly affected by Alzheimer's disease. The areas labeled include:

---

[546] Nesselroade, J. R. (2010) Methods in the study of life-span human development: Issues and answers. In W. F. Overton (Ed)., *Biology, cognition and methods across the life-span. Volume 1 of the Handbook of life-span development* (pp. 36-55), Editor-in-chief: R. M. Lerner. Hoboken, NJ: Wiley.

- Frontal lobes governing intelligence, judgment and social behavior
- Temporal lobes that process memory
- Parietal lobes that process language

It is important to point out that not all memory loss is AD. We all misplace our keys once in a while. However, memory loss that disrupts everyday life is not a typical part of aging. Normal aging produces similar changes, just not to the extent of those produced by AD. The following chart comes from The Alzheimer's Association. It illustrates these differences.[547]

| Signs of Alzheimer's Disease | Typical *Age-Related* Changes |
|---|---|
| Poor judgment and decision-making | Making a bad decision once in a while |
| Inability to manage a budget | Missing a monthly payment |
| Losing track of the date or a season | Forgetting what day it is, but remembering later |
| Difficulty maintaining a conversation | Occasionally forgetting which word to use |
| Misplacing things and being unable to retrace steps to find them | Losing things from time to time |

[547] Alzheimer's Association (2010) Alzheimer's Disease Facts and Figures. Retrieved from:
http://www.alz.org/alzheimers_disease_facts_figures.asp

## Neurotherapy and Memory Loss

In our experience, neurotherapy can be a very effective treatment for memory loss. Like physical fitness, brain fitness can be improved by disciplined exercise that presents a variety of challenges in a constructive environment. Recent research shows that regular brain "workouts" not only help prevent age-related cognitive decline, dementia, Alzheimer's and other cognitively degenerative diseases, but can even improve normally functioning minds. Although puzzles and games like chess provide mental stimulation, when it comes to improving memory, a program that challenges multiple skills in a cross-training approach has been shown to produce dramatic gains in memory capacity.

Science has shown that while genetics play a role in determining our intellectual ability (capacity), they do not limit our brains' ability to grow and change throughout our lives. Cognitive and memory programs are specifically designed to increase memory as well as intellectual abilities in a comprehensive way so our learning capacity can continue to grow and improve our overall brain function.

HEG neurofeedback helps create new neurons and connections between the neurons to enhance overall brain function. But once you've created these new connections you must exercise these connections to keep them. Especially those with degenerative types of memory loss as with Alzheimer's disease, if you don't do something with the new connections they will just die off. For this reason it is important to use other therapies such as cognitive and memory training, Neuromotor skills training, sound therapy and even audio/visual entrainment. We find that our patients with age-related memory loss can regain their abilities to recall memories in a short period of time.

## CINDY'S STORY

*Cindy is a 60 year-old female. She started losing her memory and becoming confused 10 years ago. She stopped working at her job at a delicatessen when she was unable to remember how to clean the meat slicer she had used for years.*

*Cindy's husband had read everything he could on memory loss and Alzheimer's disease. He had made sure she had all amalgams taken out of her teeth to avoid any further heavy metal contamination. He took her to Mexico twice for stem cell therapy with little effect.*

*When Cindy came to see us, she had already been diagnosed with dementia, cerebral atrophy, and neurological neglect syndrome. She had cortical blindness which affected her sight frontally, but she still had peripheral vision. Previous testing had determined that there was nothing actually wrong with her eyes, only the connections in the brain.*

*Cindy also required guidance while walking. She could not determine where doorways were located; her husband commented that he and she could no longer go to swap meets, a previously favorite activity, as she tended to wander off.*

*We assessed Cindy using a qEEG brain Map, blood oxygen levels using HEG in the frontal lobes, neuromotor skills testing and questionnaires. Our range of computer-*

*based assessments proved useless, as she was unable to see the computer screen directly in front of her.*

*Cindy appeared quite confused and was unable to follow simple instructions. Our testing for neuromotor function was very difficult for her as she was unable to locate her body in space. When clapping her hands, she would put them together and then not be able to pull them apart. When clapping one hand against her leg she would wave her hand in front of her unable to determine where her leg was.*

*HEG showed a marked decrease in activity on the right side. The results of the initial qEEG were compared to others of her age. The qEEG indicated excessive delta and theta activity in the Absolute Power calculations. Theta was also above the norm by standard deviations in the Relative Power calculations. A power asymmetry was apparent with greater power right frontally than at the left hemisphere in Delta, Theta and Alpha frequencies. Hyper-coherence or excessive communication was exhibited at occipital sites indicating lack of functional integrity at these areas. Her discriminate scores suggested Primary Degenerative Dementia.*

*We trained Cindy for a total of 20 sessions. Since we were unable to use the computer initially, we started with HEG neurofeedback at Fp1, Fp2 and Fpz. We also used audio/visual entrainment, neuromotor skills training and auditory retraining.*

*During the course of her first 10 sessions, Cindy did well. She was smiling more and able to hold a conversation. She began to clap her hands together without help and clap her hand to her leg without assistance. By the tenth session, she could see the moving landscapes on the computer screen. By the 14th session, she completed a computer-based brain speed test with some assistance. We used the visual flash for Go/No-Go testing. She was able to see the flashing figure and respond with the space bar. We used the auditory testing for digits and alphabetical characters with some help with typing. She continued to make good progress. On the 18th session her husband stated that for the first time in years, she sat down and wrote some letters. He cried.*

*At the end of 20 sessions, an additional qEEG was performed. A noticeable improvement in Power Asymmetry was noted. That is, the hemispheres were more balanced in the Delta and Theta frequencies.*

*Her behavior was noted to be more alert. Additionally, Beta hyper-coherence improved occipitally. Her motor skills improved dramatically from the first assessment. She no longer needed help to clap her hands or find her body. She was doing well on the cognitive software and could remember four to five number strings easily. Her HEG oxygen baselines steadily improved. She had a 5-7% average gain on each of the three sites every day. She was able to walk without guidance and pass through doorways without bumping into the door frames.*

*Cindy returned home to the Midwest after training. She continues to do well and is continuing her training at home.*

# CHAPTER 14
# DEPRESSION AND
# ANXIETY

Life is full of emotions. Most of us experience feelings of joy and sadness. However, constant, ongoing depression can be extremely difficult to live with, as the cause can be very hard to pinpoint.

Although the term Depression is an invention of psychiatry, the use of the term is pervasive in medicine, the media and psychology. It has become a medical diagnosis that is equated with "mood disorder" and is a collection of symptoms rather than a single illness.[548]

Depression can appear as an all-encompassing low feeling accompanied by low self-esteem and loss of interest or pleasure that hangs on for weeks. If it becomes more intense or begins to interfere with daily activities, then it is a more serious problem. It is estimated that 20 million people in the Unites States have depression. [549] Symptoms of depression can vary, but typical symptoms include:

---

[548] Gislason, S. (2010) *Human Brain in Health and Disease*. Vancouver, BC : Environmed Research Gleitman, H., Fridlund, A. J. & Reisberg, D. (2004) *Psychology* (6 ed). New York: W. W. Norton
[549] National Institute of Mental Health (2010) Depression. Retrieved from:
http://www.nimh.nih.gov/health/publications/depression/complete-index.shtml

- Agitation, restlessness, and irritability
- Dramatic changes in appetite, possibly accompanied by weight gain or loss
- Extreme difficulty concentrating
- Fatigue and lack of energy
- Feelings of guilt, hopelessness and helplessness
- Feelings of worthlessness, self-hate, and inappropriate guilt
- Loss of interest or pleasure in usual activities, or activities that were once enjoyed (such as sex)
- Thoughts of death or suicide
- Insomnia or excessive sleeping
- Persistent aches or pains, headaches, cramps or digestive problems that do not ease even with treatment

Not everyone who has depression has all these symptoms and these also vary between, men, women, children and seniors. Conversely, not everyone with some of these symptoms has depression. Depression can occur at any age. However, statistics show that depression occurs more often in women than men, through stress, loss of a loved one, hormonal changes or traumatic events.[550]

There are several types of depression including:

- Major Depressive Disorder, also called Major Depression
- Dysthymic Disorder

---

[550] Hays, R.D., Wells ,K.B. & Sherbourne, C.D. (1995) Functioning and well-being outcomes of patients with depression compared with chronic general medical illnesses. *Archives of General Psychiatry*. 1995: *52* (1), 11–19. PMID 7811158

- Psychotic Depression
- Post-Partum Depression
- Seasonal Affective Disorder
- Bipolar Disorder

The most common of these types are Major Depressive Disorder and Dysthymic Disorder.

Major Depressive Disorder is also labeled recurrent depressive disorder, clinical depression, major depression, unipolar depression, or unipolar disorder. [551] This type of depression can occur just once, but more often it is a reoccurring illness. It can be debilitating and prevent a person from normal function and enjoying life.

Impaired concentration, memory, and attention are also seen with this type of depression.[552] Research has shown that these mild cognitive abnormalities are more pronounced in those who have Major Depressive Disorder with melancholic or psychotic symptoms and who are over age 55 with signs of vascular injury to the brain.[553],[554] While the majority of studies have found these cognitive abnormalities, some studies in adults

[551] American Psychiatric Association, (2000) Diagnostic and Statistical Manual of Mental Disorders DSM-IV-TR (Fourth Edition (Text Revision) ed. Arlington, VA: American Psychiatric Publishing, Inc.
[552] Sheline YI. (2003) Neuroimaging studies of mood disorder effects on the brain. *Biol Psychiatry.* 54, 338-352.
[553] Austin, M. P., Ross, M., Murray, C., et al. (1992) Cognitive function in major depression. *J Affect Disord.* 1992 (25), 21-29.
[554] Rothschild, A.J,, Benes ,F., Hebben, N., et al. (1989) Relationships between brain CT scan findings and cortisol in psychotic and nonpsychotic depressed patients. *Biol Psychiatry, 26,*565-575.

younger than 50 years have found only mild abnormalities or normal cognitive function.[555]

In 2008, in a large European study of 8229 younger (average age, 48 years) outpatients with Major Depressive Disorder, about 2.5% were classified as normal or better than normal on a delayed recall memory test; 15.5% were rated as mildly impaired, 41% as mildly to moderately impaired, 35% as moderately to severely impaired, and only 6% as severely impaired.[556]

It is important to note that although it is common for people with Major Depressive Disorder to have a decreased ability to focus, pay attention and to have some memory loss, the magnitude of these abnormalities are still less than those found in patients with dementia, bipolar disorder, or schizophrenia.[557]

Dysthymic Disorder or as it is sometimes called Dysthymia, has less severe symptoms than Major Depressive Disorder, but it is usually long-term (more than two years) and can also prevent someone from functioning normally and enjoying life.[558] Dysthymia is

---

[555] Grant, M. M., Thase, M. E. & Sweeney, J. A. (2001) Cognitive disturbance in outpatient depressed younger adults: evidence of modest impairment. Biol Psychiatry, 50, 5-43.

[556] Gorwood , P., Corruble, E., Falissard, B. & Goodwin, G. M. (2008) Toxic effects of depression on brain function:impairment of delayed recall and the cumulative length of depressive disorder in a large sample of depressed outpatients. *Am J Psychiatry. 165*, 731-739.

[557] Zakzanis, K. K., Leach, L. & Kaplan, E. (1998) On the nature and pattern of neurocognitive function in major depressive disorder. *Neuropsychiatry Neuropsychol Behav Neurol. 11*, 111-119.

[558] Arnow, B.A., et al. (2003) Effectiveness of Psychotherapy and Combination Treatment for Chronic Depression, *Journal of Clinical Psychology , 59 (* 8), 893–905.

not a "minor" depression and it is about as common as major depression.[559] It usually identified by having at least two of the following symptoms:

- Poor appetite or overeating
- Insomnia or excessive sleep
- Low energy or fatigue
- Low self-esteem
- Poor concentration or indecisiveness
- Hopelessness

Given its chronic nature, this type of depression is most often seen by psychotherapists. About 6% of the population of the United States has had an episode of dysthymia at some time, 3% in the last year.[560]

Dysthymia most likely has a hereditary component as it appears to run in families.[561] The rate of depression in the families of those with dysthymia is as high as 50% for the early-onset form of the disorder.[562]

## CAUSES OF DEPRESSION

Depression can be caused by genetic susceptibility, neurochemical imbalances, childhood and adult stress and trauma, and social circumstances, as with isolation

---

[559] Griffiths, J., et al. (2000) Dysthymia: A Review of Pharmacological and Behavioral Factors, *Molecular Psychiatry* . 5 (3), 242–61.
[560] Klein, D. N., et al. (2003) Dysthymia and Chronic Depression: Introduction, Classification, Risk Factors, and Course, *Journal of Clinical Psychology, 59*(8), 807–16.
[561] Griffiths, J., et al. (2000) Dysthymia: A Review of Pharmacological and Behavioral Factors, *Molecular Psychiatry* . 5 (3), 242–61.
[562] Arnow, B.A., et al. (2003) Effectiveness of Psychotherapy and Combination Treatment for Chronic Depression, *Journal of Clinical Psychology* , *59 (* 8), 893–905.

and the unavailability of help.[563] Many symptoms of depression are also typical of common food-related diseases including diabetes, atherosclerosis, malnutrition, hormonal dysfunction and delayed pattern food allergy.[564] All of these problems require diet revision, but few physicians investigate this potential cause of the symptoms.

Typically, antidepressant drugs are prescribed and, if the food-related diseases are really the cause, they add to the dysfunctional chemical mix that may exist. If the first antidepressant doesn't work because of misdiagnosis, typically a second antidepressant is prescribed.

This may continue through a series of prescriptions until the patient can pause finally and examine his or her experience. At that time, most patients who have been misdiagnosed either stop taking the drugs altogether or search for a saner solution.

Most drugs prescribed for depression are SSRI's (Selective Serotonin Reuptake Inhibitors).[565] These work by preventing neurons from reabsorbing some of the "feel good" neurotransmitter, serotonin, back into the cells during inter-neuron communication. In this

---

[563] American Psychiatric Association, (2000) Diagnostic and Statistical Manual of Mental Disorders DSM-IV-TR (Fourth Edition (Text Revision) ed. Arlington, VA: American Psychiatric Publishing, Inc.
[564] Gislason, S. (2010) *Human Brain in Health and Disease*. Vancouver, BC : Environmed Research Gleitman, H., Fridlund, A. J. & Reisberg, D. (2004) *Psychology* (6 ed). New York: W. W. Norton
[565] FDA (2007) FDA Proposes New Warnings About Suicidal Thinking, Behavior in Young Adults Who Take Antidepressant Medications; *2007* (05),02.

way, the system is flooded with it, thus making the patient feel better in the short run.

With an excess of serotonin, however, the system adjusts to rebalance itself by reducing production. The excess of serotonin also can cause some adverse changes in a patient's behavior, such as increased anger, loss of libido and blunted feelings.

If the patient stops taking the medication because of these unpleasant effects, there is a secondary effect from the sudden removal of serotonin. Now he is worse off than before taking the medication; his serotonin levels are seriously out-of-balance and depression can even worsen as a result. The FDA has placed black box warnings on antidepressants because of suicidal thinking and behavior in young adults who took the drugs. [291]

## NUTRITION AND DEPRESSION

We know that depression is usually linked to stress or loss. But nutrition can also play a part. Depression may cause some to eat more while others eat less. But in both cases, it is likely that most won't maintain a healthy diet. After all, fast food, heavy in carbohydrates, acts as comfort food for most. However, sustaining healthy food is needed to maintain stable blood sugar levels. Although the brain needs glucose to enable it to perform effectively, foods high in sugars cause blood sugar levels to shoot up and then plummet, leading to lethargy. This can trigger another sweet craving, and the cycle repeats.

## ESSENTIAL FATS -OMEGA 3 (ETHYL-EPA)

Adding essential oils such as Omega 3s to the diet have been found to be very effective for depressive disorders. There have been several double-blind placebo controlled trials and in the majority of these, patients have shown significant improvement. [566],[567],[568],[569],[570] In 1999, Dr. Andrew Stoll, from Harvard Medical School, completed a study with 40 depressed patients. They were given either an omega 3 supplement or a placebo. Those given the omega 3 were found to have highly significant improvements in bipolar depression.[571],[572]

Another study, published in 2002 in the *American Journal of Psychiatry*, included twenty people suffering

[566] Hibbeln, J.R. (1998) Fish consumption and major depression. *Lancet, 351*(9110), 1213.

[567] Jazayeri ,S., Tehrani-Doost, M., Keshavarz ,S.A. et al. (2008) Comparison of therapeutic effects of omega-3 fatty acid eicosapentaenoic acid and fluoxetine, separately and in combination, in major depressive disorder. *Aust N Z J Psychiatry. 42*, 192-8.

[568] Peet, M., Horrobin, D. F. (2002) A dose-ranging study of the effects of ethyleicosapentaenoate in patients with ongoing depression despite apparently adequate treatment with standard drugs. *Arch Gen Psychiatry. 2002* (59), 913-919.

[569] Peet, M. (2003) Eicosapentaenoic acid in the treatment of schizophrenia and depression: rationale and preliminary double-blind clinical trial results. *Prostaglandins Leukot Essent Fatty Acids. 2003*(69), 477-485.

[570] Su KP, Huang SY, Chiu CC, et al. (2003) Omega-3 fatty acids in major depressive disorder—a preliminary double-blind, placebo-controlled trial. *Eur Neuropsychopharmacol. 2003* (13), 267-271.

[571] Stoll, A., Severus, W. E., Freeman, M.P., Rueter, S., Zboyan, H.A., Diamon, E., et al. (1999) Omega 3 Fatty Acids in Bipolar Disorder: A Preliminary Double-blind, Placebo-Controlled Trial . *Arch Gen Psychiatry. 1999* (56), 407-412.

[572] Stoll, A. L. (2002) The Omega-3 Connection: The Groundbreaking Antidepression Diet and Brain Program. NY: Simon & Schuster.

from severe depression who were on anti-depressants but were still exhibiting symptoms of depression. A highly concentrated form of omega 3 fat, called ethyl-EPA was tested versus a placebo. By the third week the depressed patients on the omega 3 were showing major improvements in their mood, while those on the placebo were not.[573]

In 2006, Dr Sophia Frangou of the Institute of Psychiatry studied 26 depressed people with bipolar disorder (manic depression). They administered a concentrated form of omega 3 (EPA) versus a placebo. Once again, they found a significant improvement in those depressed participants who took the omega 3.[574]

In 2006, *The Journal of Clinical Psychiatry* released a study to determine if the available data supported the use of omega 3 essential fatty acids (EFA) for clinical use in the prevention and/or treatment of psychiatric disorders. They found omega 3 EFA intake, particularly eicosapentaenoic acid (EPA) and docosahexaenoic acid (DHA), had a statistically significant benefit in unipolar and bipolar depression.[575]

---

[573] Emsley, R., Myburgh, C., Oosthuizen, P. & van Rensburg, S. J. (2002) Randomized, Placebo-Controlled Study of Ethyl-Eicosapentaenoic Acid as Supplemental Treatment in Schizophrenia . *Am J Psychiatry 159*, 1596-1598.

[574] Frangou, S., Lewis, M. & McCrone, P. (2006) Efficacy of ethyl-eicosapentaenoic acid in bipolar depression: randomised double-blind placebo-controlled study. *The British Journal of Psychiatry 188*, 46-50. doi: 10.1192/bjp.188.1.46

[575] Freeman, M.P., Hibbeln, J.R., Wisner, K.L., Davis, J.M., Mischoulon, D, Peet, M, et al. (2006) Omega-3 fatty acids: evidence basis for treatment and future research in psychiatry. *Journal of Clinical Psychiatry.* 67(12),1954–67. doi:10.4088/JCP.v67n1217. PMID 17194275

Omega 3s are found in high concentrations in oily fish such as salmon, herring, mackerel, anchovies and sardines, as well as flax seeds and walnuts-all generally considered "healthy" additions to the diet.

## B-VITAMINS

The relationship between low levels of vitamin B-12 and other B-vitamins, such as folate, also play a role in depression.[576] Although Vitamin B-12 is absent in plants, it is present in all animal tissues and is abundant in liver, kidney, other organ meats and fish. Many micro-organisms are also capable of synthesizing vitamin B-12. Though B-12 is also present in milk and dairy products, the concentration is not sufficient to meet the daily requirement.

The production of some neurotransmitters is affected by these vitamins and is important in regulating mood and other brain functions. Neurological symptoms are often the major concern regarding B-12 deficiency. The damage can be irreversible if not caught early enough.[577]

In 2008, Researchers at the Jean Mayer USDA Human Nutrition Research Center on Aging (HNRCA) at Tufts University used an experimental model to examine the metabolic, cognitive, and microvascular effects of dietary B-vitamin deficiency. Using mice, the

---

[576] Taylor, M. J. et al. (2003) Folate for depressive disorders. The Cochrane Database of Systematic Reviews 2: CD003390. DOI: 10.1002/14651858.CD003390.

[577] Scalabrino G. Subacute (2001) combined degeneration one century later. The neurotrophic action of cobalamin (vitamin B12) revisited. *J Neuropathol Exp Neurol. 60* (2), 109-20.

researchers found metabolic impairments caused by a B-vitamin (folate, B-12 and B-6) deficient diet. The deficiency caused cognitive dysfunction and reductions in brain capillary length and density in the mouse model.[578]

In 2003, researchers from the Kuopio University Hospital in Finland monitored 115 outpatients suffering from depression over a six-month period. The researchers measured blood levels of vitamin B-12 at baseline and again at the patients' six-month checkup to calculate whether the vitamin influenced patient outcome. They grouped participants according to how well they responded to treatment. The patients who responded fully to treatment had higher concentrations of vitamin B-12 in their blood at both the start and the end of the study than those, for whom treatment was less effective.[579]

## SEROTONIN LEVELS

Serotonin is an inhibitory neurotransmitter which helps us to be calm. It is made in the body and brain from an amino acid 5-Hydroxy Tryptophan (5-HTP), which is made from another amino acid called tryptophan. 5-HTP differs from tryptophan in that it

---

[578] Troen et al. (2008) B-vitamin deficiency causes hyperhomocysteinemia and vascular cognitive impairment in mice. *Proceedings of the National Academy of Sciences, 105*(34), 12474. DOI:10.1073/pnas.0805350105

[579] Hintikka, J., Tolmunen, T., Tanskanen, A. & Viinamaki, H. (2003) High vitamin B12 level and good treatment outcome may be associated in major depressive disorder *BMC Psychiatry, 3*, 17. Retrieved from: http://www.biomedcentral.com/1471-244X/3/17/abstract

slightly increases the activity of an energizing neurotransmitter, norepinephrine, as well as the calming one, serotonin.[580]

In some clinical trials, 5-HTP outperformed tryptophan in treating mood disorders. [581] Both can be found in the diet; tryptophan in many protein rich foods such as meat, fish, beans and eggs. Just not getting enough tryptophan is likely to make you depressed; people fed food deficient in tryptophan rapidly became depressed within hours.[582] Research suggests there is a deficiency of serotonin or serotonin activity in the brains of most depressed persons. [306] Suicidal patients show a significant decrease in serotonin levels.[583] Exercise, sunlight and reducing stress levels also tend to promote serotonin.[584]

## BLOOD SUGAR BALANCE

There is a direct link between mood and blood sugar balance. All carbohydrate foods are broken down into glucose which fuels your brain. The more uneven your blood sugar supply, the more uneven your mood.[585]

---

[580] Baumel, S. (1995) Dealing with Depression Naturally. CT :Keats.

[581] Baumel, S. (1997) Serotonin: How to Naturally Harness the Power Behind Prozac and Phen/Fen. CT: Keats.

[582] Schaechter, J.D., Wurtman ,R.J. (1990) Serotonin release varies with brain tryptophan levels. *Brain Res.* 532(1-2), 203–10. doi:10.1016/0006-8993(90)91761-5.

[583] Braverman, E. (1997) *The Healing Nutrients Within*. CT: Keats.

[584] Young, S. (2007) How to increase serotonin in the human brain without drugs. *J Psychiatry Neurosci.* 2007 November, *32*(6), 394–399.

[585] National Institute of Mental Health (2010) Depression. Retrieved from:
http://www.nimh.nih.gov/health/publications/depression/complete-index.shtml

Sugar can give you rapid changes in the level of blood glucose. Symptoms can include

- Fatigue
- Irritability
- Dizziness
- Insomnia
- Night sweats
- Poor concentration and forgetfulness
- Excessive thirst
- Depression and crying spells
- Digestive disturbances
- Blurred vision

Since the brain depends on an even supply of glucose it is no surprise to find that sugar has been implicated in aggressive behavior, anxiety, depression and fatigue.[586]

## CHROMIUM

Chromium is a mineral that is vital for maintaining stable blood sugar level because insulin, which clears glucose from the blood, can't work properly without it. In fact, it turns out that just supplying proper levels of chromium to certain depressed patients can make a significant difference.[587]

Atypical depression, a subtype of dysthymia and major depression, shares many of the symptoms of both, but

---

[586] Fittante, A. (2006) The Sugar Solution: Weight Gain? Memory Lapses? Mood Swings? Fatigue? Your Symptoms Are Real — And Your Solution is Here. CA: Rodale Books.
[587] Rabinovitz, H., Friedensohn, A., Leibovitz, A., Gabay ,G., Rocas, C. & Habot, B. (2004) Effect of chromium supplementation on blood glucose and lipid levels in type 2 diabetes mellitus elderly patients. *Int J Vitam Nutr Res.*, 74 (3), 178-82.

also is characterized by mood reactivity-being able to experience an improved mood in response to positive events. Dr. Malcolm McLeod, clinical professor of psychiatrist at the University of North Carolina, suggests that people who suffer with "atypical" depression might benefit from chromium supplementation.

In a small double-blind study, McLeod gave 600mcg chromium supplements daily to ten patients suffering from atypical depression gave placebos to five others. This study was conducted over an eight-week period. The results were dramatic. Seven of ten taking the supplements showed a significant improvement, versus none on the placebo. McLeod used the Hamilton Rating Score for depression to measure symptoms in his patients. The scores of those on chromium dropped by 83%; from 29 (major depression) to five (not depressed). [588]

A larger trial at Cornell University with 113 patients has confirmed McLeod's findings. After eight weeks, 65% of those on chromium had experiences a major improvement, compared to 33% on placebos.[589]

## THOUGHTS AFFECT DEPRESSION

Another area seldom discussed in depression patients is their ability to bring themselves down so profoundly

---

[588] McLeod, M.L. (2005) *Lifting Depression: The Chromium Connection.* Chapel Hill, NC : Basic Health Publications.
[589] Docherty, J.P, et al. (2005) Chromium and Depression. *Journal of Psychiatric Practice, 11* (5), 302.

with their own thoughts. Our thoughts can actually influence how we feel.[590]

Depression is exacerbated by negative thoughts and our reaction to stress. [591] When we are depressed we generally ruminate on the negatives in our lives such as "I don't feel good" or "I'm never going to feel good" or "everything is bad". Those negative thoughts could, in fact, be the cause of the problem!

The average person has many thousands of thoughts each day. If one's state of mind is predominantly negative, imagine how many negative thoughts are generated daily. It's clear that depression causes negative thoughts, but can negative thoughts cause depression? The answer might lie in the fact that humans mistakenly see their thoughts as privileged communication, occupying a rarefied space, immune to mood and feelings, and so represent some incontrovertible truth. Therefore the negative thoughts we allow ourselves to think seem harmless. We are unaware that the despair and hopelessness we feel may actually be coming from our negative thoughts. If left unchecked, our negative thoughts can actually cause physical changes, such as negative eating and sleeping patterns or even psychotic changes such as hallucinations and delusions. To make matters worse, we generate negative thoughts so automatically we are

---

[590] Salovey, P. & Birnbaum, D. (1989) Influence of mood on health-relevant cognitions. *Journal of Personality and Social Psychology. 57*(3), 539-551. doi: 10.1037/0022-3514.57.3.539
[591] Gunthert, K.C., Cohen, L.H., Butler A.C. &Beck, J.S. (2007) Depression and Next-day Spillover of Negative Mood and Depressive Cognitions Following Interpersonal Stress . *Journal of Cognitive Therapy and Research, 31*, 4. DOI: 10.1007/s10608-006-9074-1

unaware that they are happening. Negative thinking is one of the strongest habit patterns.[592]

Understanding how our thinking affects our health is one of the most powerful actions we can take in combating depression. Often we can't control how we feel, but we can control how we think. It's an active choice we can make—if we are aware that changing our thinking is important.

If you still have doubts that our thoughts affect everything in and around us, Masaru Emoto, a creative and visionary Japanese researcher has findings that may interest you. He has been researching how thought affects water. Considering that water comprises over seventy percent of a mature human body, his results are directly related to how thoughts affect us.[593]

Mr. Emoto has been visually documenting molecular changes in water which have been exposed to human vibrational energy, thoughts, words, ideas and music by means of his photographic techniques. He freezes droplets of water and then examines them under a dark field microscope with photographic capabilities. His photos remind us that we can change ourselves and the world we live in just with our thoughts. These images are evidence of our innate ability to heal and transform ourselves by the thoughts we choose to think and the ways we put those thoughts into action.

---

[592] Mayo Clinic (2010) Positive thinking: Reduce stress, enjoy life more. Retrieved from: http://www.mayoclinic.com/health/positive-thinking/sr00009
[593] Emoto, Masaru (2004) *The Hidden Messages in Water*. Hillsboro, OR: Beyond Words Publishing.

## TIPS TO CHANGE THINKING PATTERNS

One of the most powerful actions we can take in combating depression is to understand how critical the quality of our thinking is to maintaining and even intensifying depression—and that the quickest way to change how we feel is to change how we think.[594]

Here are some tips and hints on depression and how to get rid of it.

- Know that it is possible for you to change how you think. It will help change how you feel more than anything. Remember, it's not changing how you feel so you will think more positively. It is the other way around.
- Keep track of your negative thoughts. Do this for two or three days to see just how often during the day your thoughts turn negative.
- Keep a journal of all your negative thoughts for several days. If you can't write a thought down every time you have one, take time at the end of the day to go over your thoughts and write them down. Did you think, "I'm too fat, lazy, stupid, careless?" Even include messages to self: "I hate my job, my life, my boss." Also include those times in which you call yourself a name such as "idiot," or think of yourself (or someone else) as worthless.

---

[594] Marano, H.E. (2001) Depression Doing the Thinking .*Psychology Today*. Retrieved from: http://www.psychologytoday.com/articles/200308/depression-doing-the-thinking

- Make sure you note any negative thinking focused on a problem rather than on solutions. Jot down when you feel you're a victim, even if it's legitimate.
- Keep track of those times when you feel helpless or hopeless. Be particularly aware of making generalizations from one specific bad event so that your whole future appears to be terrible. "I got fired from this job; I'll never have a good job again." "This relationship broke up; I'll never find a partner." Listen for words that are categorical and extreme-always, never. Black-and-white thinking is another sign-it's usually too extreme.
- Alternatively to keeping a journal, carry with you a stack of index cards, a smart phone or a small computer and note negative thoughts as they occur. Although describing the negative thoughts is more helpful, it is not essential; you can simply tally them.
- Develop a partnership strategy. Ask a loved one or a trusted colleague to point out your instances of negative thinking, and then record them.
- After you see the kind of negative thinking and its frequency, identify the situations that trigger such thinking. The act of writing down instances of negative thinking is an exercise that helps make you aware of your triggers.
- Change negative to positive thinking the next time you encounter a trigger. Just flip the switch.
- It helps to have a visual reminder. Keep a sign or an object you have designated for this purpose. Refer to it often to remind you when you slip.
- Remember to be aware. When you catch yourself saying or thinking something negative. Stop yourself and rephrase to make your intent positive.

Change, "I'm too fat." To be "I've been fat before but now I'm working hard at being fit." Even if you don't believe it! This will help your brain to start focusing on the positive things around you.

- Have friends and relatives help you. Tell your mate or trusted colleague that you think you're sounding too pessimistic in your thinking and that you want to be more optimistic; ask them to help you out by giving you a cue

## DEPRESSION AND NEUROTHERAPY

Neurotherapy has been very successful with those who have depression and anxiety.[595], [596],[597] Neurotherapy lets the patient exert control over involuntary muscle and brain activities by training the brain to react to its own signals. This treatment has been shown to be effective for relieving symptoms of depression and anxiety.

---

[595] Davidson, R. J. (1998) Affective style and affective disorders: Perspectives from affective
neuroscience. *Cognition & Emotion, 12*, 307-330.
[596] Davidson, R. J. (1998) Anterior electrophysiological asymmetries, emotion, and depression: Conceptual and methodological conundrums. *Psychophysiology, 35*, 607-614.
[597] Hammond, D. C. (2000). Neurofeedback treatment of depression with the Roshi. *Journal of Neurotherapy*, 4(2), 45-56.

## The Limbic System

The limbic system of the brain has been recognized as a central area involved in depression and anxiety.[598] It regulates activities such as, emotions, physical and sexual drives as well as stress. The hypothalamus, a small structure located at the base of the brain, is responsible for many basic functions such as body temperature, sleep, appetite, sexual drive, stress reaction, and the regulation of other activities. The hypothalamus also controls the function of the pituitary gland which in turn regulates key hormones. Other structures within the limbic system that are associated with emotional reaction are the amygdala and hippocampus. The activities of the limbic are so important and complex that disturbances in any part of it, including how neurotransmitters function, could affect mood and behavior.[599]

## Neurotransmitters and Neurons

Neurotransmitters, the special chemicals that help transfer messages throughout structures of the brain's nerve cells, are called upon whenever we react or feel emotions. Our neurons transmit messages in the form

---

[598] Ito, H., Kawashima, R., Awata, S., Ono, S., Sato,K., Goto, R. et al. (1996) Hypoperfusionin the Limbic System and Prefrontal Cortex in Depression: SPECT with Anatomic Standardization Technique. Department of Nuclear Medicine and Radiology, Division of Brain Sciences, Institute of Development, Aging and Cancer, Tohoku University, and Department of Psychiatry, Tohoku University School of Medicine, Sendai, Japan. Retrieved from:: jnm.snmjournals.org/cgi/reprint/37/3/410.pdf
[599] Morgan, L. O. (1939) Alterations in the Hypothalamus in Mental Deficiency. *Psychosomatic Medicine, 1,4.*

of electrical impulses from one cell to another. These electrical impulses travel across the neurons at an amazing rate of speed—less than 1/5,000 of a second. Because they move so quickly, our brains can react instantaneously to stimuli such as pain.[600]

Of the 30 or so neurotransmitters that have been identified, researchers have discovered associations between clinical depression and the function of three primary ones: serotonin, norepinephrine, and dopamine. These three neurotransmitters function within structures of the brain that regulate emotions, reactions to stress, and the physical drives of sleep, appetite, and sexuality.[601]

It is unknown whether changes in levels of neurotransmitters cause the development of depression or depression causes changes in neurotransmitters. It may happen both ways. Researchers believe that our behavior can affect our brain chemistry, and that brain chemistry can affect behavior. For instance, if a person experiences numerous stressors or traumas this may cause his or her brain chemistry to be affected, leading to clinical depression. On the other hand, that same person may learn how to change depressed thoughts and behavior and cope with stressful events. Doing this may also change brain chemistry and relieve depression.[602]

---

[600] Saladin, K. S. (2010) *Anatomy & Physiology Fifth Edition*. Columbus, OH: McGraw Hill.

[601] Rang, H. P. (2003) *Pharmacology*. Edinburgh: Churchill Livingstone.

[602] University of Bristol (2009) Introduction to Serotonin. Retrieved from: http://www.chm.bris.ac.uk/motm/serotonin/introduction.htm

Neurotherapy can affect depression without medications. It lets you have control over how your brain reacts and how it uses the neurotransmitters. Neurotherapies can calm the limbic system, relieving the "fight or flight" response and alleviating stress.[603]

An area in the limbic system called the nucleus accumbens is the reward center of the brain.[604] Stimulation of this area using neurotherapy has shown reductions in depressed mood while also increasing the capacity for pleasure. [605] Neurofeedback stimulates this area to reduce feelings of depression and enhance the feeling of wellbeing.

## OUR CLINICAL EXPERIENCE

In our experience, neurofeedback training appears to be effective regardless of the reason a person has become depressed. It could be a genetic pre-disposition, early childhood trauma, a traumatic (physical or emotional) experience, or simply an unknown physiological change. If a client is taking an antidepressant medication at the start of training, he may find that during training he may be able to cut back on medication or stop it altogether. For this reason, we insist that a person taking psychotropic

---

[603] Schaechter, J.D., Wurtman ,R.J. (1990) Serotonin release varies with brain tryptophan levels. *Brain Res. 532*(1-2), 203–10. doi:10.1016/0006-8993(90)91761-5.
[604] Schwienbacher I., Fendt, M., Richardson, R. & Schnitzler, H. U. (2004) Temporary inactivation of the nucleus accumbens disrupts acquisition and expression of fearpotentiated startle in rats. *Brain Res. 1027*(1-2), 87–93. doi:10.1016/j.brainres.2004.08.037
[605] Menon, V. & Levitin, D.J. (2005) The rewards of music listening: Response and physiological connectivity of themesolimbic system. *NeuroImage 28*(1), 175-184.

medication under the supervision of a physician should always continue that professional consultation during our training so that reduction of medication can be accomplished safely. Generally we see anti-depressant medication reduced or eliminated entirely as the training proceeds and the patient is able to function normally on their own.

Sometimes depression can be accompanied by memories of prior traumatic incidents, which may have been totally suppressed over the years. In these instances counseling or hypnotherapy can be very helpful.[606] Neurotherapy has also been found to be helpful in Post-Traumatic Stress Disorder (PTSD). PTSD can be caused by specific traumatic events, such as rape, military service during wartime, being a victim of a violent act or even a witness to a violent act.[607]

There is evidence that once a person experiences depression, subsequent episodes are more likely. Therefore, neurotherapy is very helpful as it is a permanent solution and can therefore make subsequent recurrences less likely.[608] Neurotherapy also appears to be effective for a variety of conditions

---

[606] Brom, D., Kleber, R. J. & Defares, P. B. (1989) Brief psychotherapy of posttraumatic stress disorders. *J Consult Clin Psychol, 57,* 607–612.
[607] Esty, M.L. & Nelson, D. (2009) Neurotherapy of TBI/PTSD in OEF/OIF Veterans. *The Journal of Neuropsychiatry and Clinical Neurosciences, 21,* 221-223.
[608] Lane, J. D., Kasian, S. J., Owens, J. E. & Marsh, G. R. (1998) Binaural auditory beats affect vigilance performance and mood. *Physiol Behav. 63,* 249-252.

which are seen together with depression, such as addiction and violent behavior.[609],[610],[611]

## Depression and Exercise

Many depression patients are so depressed they find it hard to get up from their beds to seek help.[612] Researchers are finding that exercise may be the key to be able to help yourself. The word "exercise" may make you think of running laps around the gym, but a wide range of activities that boost your activity level can help you feel better.

Don't pump iron and lift weights—those activities have been shown to worsen anxiety. Instead, work in the garden, wash your car, or walk around the block. Anything that gets you off the couch and moving is exercise that can help improve your mood. Can't get started? Start simple. Get out your gym shorts and place them on a chair. You don't have to put them on. Do the same thing the next day and put them on. You don't have to go out and exercise. Just walk around in

[609] Wong, M.R., Brochin, N.E., & Genfron, K.L. (1981) Effects of meditation on anxiety and chemical dependency. *Journal of Drug Education, 11,* 91-105.

[610] Wahbeh, H., Calabrese, C. & Zwickey, H., (2007) Binaural beat technology in humans: a pilot study to assess psychologic and physiologic effects. *J Altern Complement Med. 13,* 25-32.

[611] Wahbeh, H., Calabrese, C., Zwickey, H. & Zajdel, D. (2007b) Binaural beat technology in humans: a pilot study to assess neuropsychologic, physiologic, and electroencephalographic effects. *J Altern Complement Med. 13,* 199-206.

[612] Babyak, M. Blumenthal, J. A., Herman, S., Khatri, P., Doraiswamy, M.,Moore, K. et al. (2000) Exercise Treatment for Major Depression: Maintenance of Therapeutic Benefit at 10 Months. *Psychosomatic Medicine, 62,*633-638.

your gym clothes. Work your way up to actually going to do that exercise.

You also don't have to do all your exercise at once. Broaden how you think of exercise and find ways to fit activity into your routine. Add small amounts of physical activity throughout your day. For example, take the stairs instead of the elevator. Next time, park a little farther away from work to fit in a short walk. Or, if you live close to your job, consider biking to work.

We've seen that doing as little as 30 minutes of exercise a day, for three to five days a week can significantly improve depression symptoms. But smaller amounts of activity—as little as 10 to 15 minutes at a time—can make a difference. Exercise probably helps ease depression because the activity is:

- Releasing feel-good brain chemicals that may ease depression (neurotransmitters and endorphins)
- Reducing immune system chemicals that can worsen depression
- Increasing body temperature, which may have calming effects

Exercise has many psychological and emotional benefits too. It can also help you:

- Gain confidence. Meeting exercise goals or challenges, even small ones, can boost your self-confidence. Getting in shape can also make you feel better about your appearance.
- Take your mind off worries. Exercise is a distraction that can get you away from the cycle of negative thoughts that feed anxiety and depression.

- Get more social interaction. Exercise may give you the chance to meet or socialize with others. Just exchanging a friendly smile or greeting as you walk around your neighborhood can help your mood.
- Cope in a healthy way. Doing something positive to manage anxiety or depression is a healthy coping strategy. Trying to feel better by drinking alcohol, dwelling on how badly you feel, or hoping anxiety or depression will go away on their own can lead to worsening symptoms.[613]

## NATHAN'S STORY

*Nathan is a 17-year-old boy who had been an enthusiastic learner in elementary school. In kindergarten he was observed once by a speech teacher, but she did not think speech was an issue. He was a little slow learning to read, but once he was in a school that used a strong phonics program, his reading ability took off. He was placed in advanced math in third grade. When Nathan was ready for junior high he was placed in a college preparatory school. He loved his 7th grade year and while he wasn't a straight-A student, his enthusiasm and eagerness to learn was obvious. He was awarded the Virtus Award by his teachers for outstanding character.*

*During the summer before his 8th grade year (2006), Nathan was at scout camp when on the last day, the troop decided to take a mountain bike ride. Near the end of the ride, Nathan's bike hit a pothole. He flew off the bike and landed on his head and right shoulder. His*

---

[613] Johnsgard, K. (2004) *Conquering Depression and Anxiety Through Exercise*. New York: Prometheus Books.

*helmet was cracked in six places. The rest of the summer he rested.*

*When he started school that August, his enthusiasm for learning was gone and he started to struggle. He now found schoolwork overwhelming. When he focused on one subject to bring a grade up another subject would slide. Eventually his doctors diagnosed him with a Traumatic Brain Injury. He started taking supplements and antidepressants; however he continued to be depressed. He struggled with reading and comprehension. He had difficulty shifting attention from one subject to another when working on homework. He passed the school year but failed 3 of 6 classes. His social life was failing as well. He had been much more social before the accident. Afterwards he had few friends and didn't enjoy a social life as he had in the past.*

*When Nathan came to see us at BrainAdvantage, he was on Celexa, tired, withdrawn and very unhappy. He started our BrainAdvantage training. After a few sessions, I asked him how he felt. His response was "Happy!" with a large smile. By the 10th session, he had been weaned off all medication. He was bright and cheerful. By the 20th session he had made remarkable improvement. His mother came in to the final evaluation. She said, "You've given me back my son." Nathan was cheerful and had started work on a novel. Life looked much better to him.*

# CHAPTER 15
# TRAUMATIC BRAIN
# INJURY

According to the Center for Disease Control (CDC), over 1. 7 million people are seen in emergency rooms for traumatic brain injury (TBI) in the United States every year. Of those 1.7 million approximately 50,000 adults and 2,685 children die; 235,000 adults and 37,000 children are hospitalized; and 1.1 million adults and 435,000 children are treated and released from an emergency department. [614],[615]

Many times, however, those who sustain a head injury are never diagnosed. Some don't report the injury and never go the emergency room. The symptoms of brain injury can be subtle and therefore ignored. Sometimes the symptoms of a TBI may not appear until days or weeks later.[616] TBI can cause a wide range of functional changes that can affect thinking, sensation, language, and/or emotions. It can also cause epilepsy and

---

[614] Center for Disease Control (2010) Injury Prevention & Control: Traumatic Brain Injury. Retrieved from:
http://www.cdc.gov/traumaticbraininjury/
[615] Finkelstein, E., Corso, P., Miller, T., et al. (2006) *The Incidence and Economic Burden of Injuries in the United States*. New York: Oxford University Press.
[616] Langlois, J.A., Rutland-Brown, W. & Thomas, K.E. (2004) Traumatic brain injury in the United States: emergency department visits, hospitalizations, and deaths. Atlanta (GA): Centers for Disease Control and Prevention, National Center for Injury Prevention and Control

increase the risk for conditions such as Alzheimer's disease, Parkinson's disease, and other brain disorders that become more prevalent with age.[617]

Here is the list of symptoms to look for according to the CDC:

- Headaches or neck pains that do not go away
- Difficulty remembering, concentrating, or making decisions
- Slower thinking, speaking, acting, or reading
- Getting lost or easily confused
- Feeling tired all of the time, having no energy or motivation
- Mood changes (feeling sad or angry for no reason)
- Changes in sleep patterns (sleeping a lot more or having a hard time sleeping)
- Light-headedness, dizziness, or loss of balance
- Urge to vomit (nausea)
- Increased sensitivity to lights, sounds, or distractions
- Blurred vision or eyes that tire easily
- Loss of sense of smell or taste
- Ringing in the ears

Often children are a little harder to diagnose with TBI as it is harder for them to let adults know how they

---

[617] Robinson, R. G. & Szetela, B. (2004) Mood change following left hemispheric brain injury. *Annals of Neurology*, 9(5), 447 – 453.

feel. Here is a list of symptoms to look for in children following a blow to the head:

- Tiredness or listlessness
- Irritability or crankiness (will not stop crying or cannot be consoled)
- Changes in eating (will not eat or nurse)
- Changes in sleep patterns
- Changes in the way the child plays
- Changes in performance at school
- Lack of interest in favorite toys or activities
- Loss of new skills, such as toilet training
- Loss of balance or unsteady walking
- Vomiting

## WHAT IS A TBI?

An acquired brain injury is damage to the brain caused by anything that would be acquired, such as tumors, strokes, or a traumatic injury.[618] Traumatic brain injury (TBI) is more specific as it implies trauma to the brain caused by the infliction of an external force upon the head and brain.[619]

---

[618] Chapman, S.B., Levin, H.S., Lawyer, S.L. (1999) Communication problems resulting from brain injury in children: Special issues of assessment and management. in McDonald, S., Togher, L., Code, C. *Communication Disorders Following Traumatic Brain Injury.* East Sussex: Psychology Press. pp. 235–36. Retrieved from: http://books.google.com/books?id=klwVAAAAIAAJ&pg=PA236&dq=no ntraumatic+%22Acquired+brain+injury&client=fi refox-a"http://books.google.com/books?id=klwVAAAAIAAJ&pg=PA236&dq= nontraumatic+%22Acquired+brain+injury&client=firefox-a.

[619] Blissitt, P. A .( 2006) Care of the critically ill patient with penetrating head injury. *Critical Care Nursing Clinics of North America, 18* (3), 321–32. doi:10.1016/j.ccell.2006.05.006. PMID 16962454

According to the National Institute of Neurological Disorders and Stroke, the brain is protected from bumps and jolts by floating in a surrounding layer of cerebral fluid. If the head suffers a severe blow or a violent jolt, the brain can bump hard against the bony outcroppings of the interior skull. This can result in the tearing of fibrous material, nerves and rupturing of blood vessels under the skull leading to an accumulation of blood. Sometimes these injuries don't even show up on an MRI.

Not all blows or jolts to the head result in a TBI. The severity of a TBI may range from "mild," i.e., a brief change in mental status or consciousness to "severe," i.e., an extended period of unconsciousness or amnesia after the injury.[620]

## CLOSED VERSUS OPEN HEAD INJURIES

A more specific way to classify TBI is closed versus open head injury.

## CLOSED HEAD INJURY

A closed head injury is a trauma in which the brain is injured as a result of a blow to the head, or a sudden, violent motion that causes the brain to knock against the skull. A closed head injury is different from an open head injury, in that no object actually penetrates the brain. Closed head injuries can be *diffuse*, meaning that they affect cells and tissues throughout the brain; or

---

[620] National Institute of Neurological Disorders & Stroke. (2002) Traumatic brain injury: hope through research. Bethesda (MD): National Institutes of Health; 2002 Feb. *NIH Publication* No.: 02–158.

*focal*, meaning that the damage occurs in one area. Closed head injuries can range from mild to severe.

Common causes of closed head injury include automobile accidents, assault, falls, work-related accidents, and sports-related accidents.

## *OPEN HEAD INJURY*

An open head injury, or a penetrating head injury, results when an object penetrates the skull and enters the brain. Open head injuries are usually *focal*. Open head injuries are very serious and can cause permanent disability, and even death.

Open head injury can be caused by high-velocity objects such as bullets, but can also be caused by low-velocity objects such as knives and other weapons. One of the most common causes of open brain injury is skull fracture, in which a piece of bone from the skull penetrates the brain. Skull fractures can be caused by a blow to the head, car accidents, a fall, or a sports or athletic injury.

## NEUROTHERAPY AND TBI

TBI disrupts connections in the neural circuitry, which can lead to damage in a specific area creating abnormal brain activity.[621] Traditional treatment for TBI not requiring surgery has been limited to medications, talk therapy and physical therapy. Depending on the

---

621 Rehman, T., Ali, R., Tawil, I. & Yonas, H. (2008) Rapid progression of traumatic bifrontal contusions to transtentorial herniation: A case report. *Cases journal* , 1(1), 203. doi:10.1186/1757-1626-1-203. PMID 18831756

severity of the injury, most traditional rehabilitation focuses on regaining the ability to socialize, overcome low self-esteem, and relearn speech and mobility. However we now know that it is also possible to reestablish the much needed communication pathways in the brain.

While these damaged areas are unlikely to repair themselves on their own, through neurotherapy other pathways can be created to take the place of those damaged. [349] Neurotherapy doesn't actively do anything to the brain; rather, it seems to stimulate the brain to change itself and to recover its natural flexibility of functioning. The brain finds its own path to optimal self-regulation. Neurofeedback is safe and its effects are long-lasting.

Neurologist Jonathan Walker, M.D., based his study of coherence neurotherapy (affecting the connections between two sites) for persons with mild closed head injuries. Twenty-six patients were seen three to seventy months after their head traumas and were given, on the average, nineteen, individualized sessions of EEG biofeedback. Greater than fifty percent improvement was seen in eighty-eight percent of the patients. All persons who had been working prior to their injury were able to return to work.[622]

---

[622] Walker, J. E., Norman, C. A., & Weber, R. (2002) Impact of QEEG-guided coherence training for patients with a mild closed head injury. *J. Neurotherapy*, 6:31-43

## Other Issues with TBI

Neurotherapy makes TBI recovery much faster and easier.[623],[624] But we know that healing or compensating for the damage to the brain is just part of the recovery for TBI patients. Many of our TBI patients report that they feel as if they were "reborn" after their accident. The old personality is gone. A new person now sits at the helm. They may look the same, but they are not the same person and that is part of the difficulty.

Once the physical side heals, others think that the injured person is back to normal. Much of the time, however, the cognitive and emotional difficulties can be even more devastating and take much longer to heal. Often the system has been sufficiently disrupted for long enough that the symptoms are not yet completely relieved. Disorganization of thoughts, problems with planning and short-term memory disturbances can continue to be an issue.

Anxious to heal, TBI patients often push themselves to try and take on those things they were doing before the accident. This can cause more problems because they have not let the brain heal. Some say they feel fatigued, as if they have been without sleep for days. They sometimes liken it to a constant meditative state.

---

[623] Duff, J. (2004) The usefulness of quantitative EEG (QEEG) and neurotherapy in the assessment and treatment of post-concussion syndrome. *Clin EEG Neurosci.*, *35* (4), 198-209.
[624] Thornton, K.E. (2000) Exploratory Analysis: Mild Head Injury, Discriminant Analysis with High Frequency Bands (32-64 Hz) under Attentional Activation Conditions & Does Time Heal?. *Journal of Neurotherapy, Feb., 2000*, 1-10.

During these times there is no inner chatter, just quiet darkness. During these times the brain is trying to heal itself and therefore goes "offline." When this happens they can be physically unable to stay connected mentally.

Counseling becomes more difficult because patients can't track everything that's being said. They don't remember conversations and often require others to re-explain things they've already been told. This is devastating to many who were used to having a smart, sharp mind and being in control. The brain fatigue that occurs with these injuries is devastating. Patients are no longer able to do all the things they did before. To make matters worse, often people in their lives don't understand the full implications of the injuries, especially those used to being cared for by the brain-injured individual. The inability of the patient to think clearly and act quickly can seem to be a personal affront to them. Perhaps this person is withholding from them purposely or faking their injuries to gain sympathy.

These reactions can be devastating to the injured patient. Not only is the patient struggling with physical problems, he or she is now stressed and frustrated, trying to explain the realities to those who are closest to them. The real absurdity is thinking that a brain-injured person will have the wherewithal to put into words the physical symptoms, anxiety, depression and frustration he or she feels. Although neurotherapy can shorten the recovery by years, it is still takes time and work to recover completely.

## Sandy's Story

*Sandy is a beautiful young woman who was a passenger in a roll-over motor vehicle accident after a friend fell asleep at the wheel. The car rolled over four times. Sandy fractured her cervical spine and suffered many cuts in her scalp. With these injuries, doctors failed to notice on first examination that Sandy had also sustained a head injury. She was left with severe headaches and neck pain, difficulty recalling and spelling words, and loss of her ability to find her way to familiar places.*

*Sandy also suffered with pain down both of her legs and "jumpy leg syndrome." She kept dropping things with her right arm and was crying every day. At the time of the accident, Sandy was serving as office manager and de facto IT manager in a multi-physician group. After the accident, Sandy was unable to find her way to the office, much less function as the office manager.*

*For four months, she received treatment at a noted neurological hospital, but with no success. Her neurologist finally told her, "Just go home and sit down. It will take you 1½ years to recover and then you'll be fine." Her husband had recommended that she come to our office but her neurologist responded, "Oh, no, don't do that. All that neurotherapy has no science. It's just experimental." Fortunately, she decided to come anyway.*

*She was driven to our office by a friend who helped her in for her first appointment. Her initial evaluation of memory showed marked decrease in both memory and executive function. Hemoencephalographic evaluation showed low activity in the right frontal lobe, the seat of spatial memory processing. Initial test of her ability to maintain focus and attention indicated that he was markedly positive for Attention Deficit Disorder.*

*She started with BrainAdvantage training three days a week. After the second session, Sandy was able to turn her cell phone volume to half what she had required when she first started therapy. After the third session, she stopped crying and was able to find her way to our office without assistance.*

*After the fifth session she reported that she had helped her son with his trigonometry homework, the first time she had been able to do that since the accident.*

*At the tenth neurotherapy session, Sandy had been weaned off all medications. Her attention test scores indicated that she was well outside the range for Attention Deficit Disorder. Her memory and executive function had improved dramatically, as had her oxygen levels in the brain.*

*Sandy had other changes resulting from the traumatic brain injury. Her personality had changed somewhat. She was no longer what she described as a "pleaser," someone who wanted to please everyone all the time. After she was able to think a little more clearly, she insisted on a mutual effort around her house. This change did not please her family. After all, they were used to her doing everything for them all the time.*

*After the 20th session, she was able to function as the office manager again, although multi-tasking was still somewhat difficult for her. Her memory had improved significantly, and she no longer had any difficulty with spatial processing.*

*It wasn't long after Sandy finished her program with us that Dr. Jill Bolte Taylor came to town to give a talk to a new women's group through A.T. Still University, an osteopathic medical school. Dr. Taylor is a Harvard-trained neuroanatomist who had suffered a stroke at the age of 37. In her amazing book, My Stroke of Insight, Dr. Taylor describes how it felt to have the stroke and brilliantly illustrates how different parts of the brain work. She also tells of her eight-year-long road to recovery.*

*You can see and hear her describe her incredible experiences at http://www.ted.com/talks/jill_bolte_taylor_s_powerful_s troke_of_insight.html*

*I took Sandy to meet Dr. Taylor. It was inspiring for Sandy to hear how others had experienced the same issues that she had after the accident. The personality change was common, according to Dr. Taylor. She told Sandy, "That Jill Taylor died the day of the stroke and this Jill Taylor was reborn."*

*Although Sandy recovered amazingly quickly, she still works on her other issues every day. She has had to accept the fact that she is a different person than she was before the accident.*

# CHAPTER 16
# ADDICTION AND
# NEUROTHERAPY

Addiction, or Substance Abuse Disorder, is a neurobiological disorder that causes a continued compulsive behavior despite detrimental effects. Although drugs and alcohol are the most commonly thought of addictions, addiction can also occur with other substances and activities as well, such as food, sex, shopping, gambling, etc.[625]

In our society, addiction impacts every community, every family and all income levels. Hundreds of billions of dollars in taxpayer money are spent each year either directly on addiction or on its devastating end results. But addiction isn't merely a social problem. It isn't limited to criminals and those with weak characters and weak minds.[626] According to the Substance Abuse and Mental Health Services Administration's (SAMHSA's) National Survey on Drug Use and Health in 2006, 23.6 million persons aged 12 or older needed treatment for an illicit drug or alcohol abuse problem (9.6 percent of the persons aged 12 or older).

---

[625] Collins, A. (2009) Neurofeedback for Addictions: The State of the Science. ISNR. Retrieved from:
http://www.isnr.org/information/addiction.cfm
[626] Sergo, P. (2008) New Weapons against Cocaine Addiction. *Scientific American Mind*, Retrieved from:
http://www.scientificamerican.com/article.cfm?id=new-weapons-against-cocaine-addiction

---

## ADDICTION AND THE BRAIN

Addiction is a disease, a chronic relapsing brain disease that severely alters those areas in the brain critical to decision making, learning, memory, and behavior control. [627] With addiction, dramatic changes to synapses are also found.[628]

By bypassing the five senses and directly activating the brain's reward circuitry, drugs can cause a jolt of intense pleasure. As the brain continues to adapt to the presence of the drug, regions outside of the reward pathway are also affected. Brain regions responsible for judgment, learning and memory begin to physically change or become "hard-wired". [629]

According to Dr. Nora Volkow, Director of the National Institute on Drug Abuse, addicted brains "have been modified by the drug in such a way that absence of the drug sends a signal to their brain that is equivalent to the signal you receive when you are starving. It acts as if the individual is in a state of deprivation and taking

---

[627] Hyman, S. E. & Malenka, R.C. (2001) Addiction and the brain: the neurobiology of compulsion and its persistence. *Nat Rev Neurosci*; 2: 695-703

[628] Lingford-Hughes, A. & Nutt, D .(2003) Neurobiology of addiction and implications for treatment. *Br J Psychiatry*, *182*, 97-100.

[629] Richards, K.L. (2010) Opioids: Addiction vs. Dependence. Retrieved from: http://www.healthcentral.com/chronic-pain/coping-279488-5.html

the drug is essential for survival. It's as powerful as that." [630]

Adolescents are especially vulnerable to addiction, as the adolescent brain is still developing, particularly in the areas of judgment and impulse control. Also, adolescents have a heightened sensitivity to social and peer pressures. As time goes on, an adolescent addiction becomes more serious.[631]

Substance abuse disorders can be measured by the amount, frequency and context of a person's substance use. As their illness deepens, addicted people need more alcohol or other drugs; they may use more often, and use it in situations they never imagined when they first began to drink or take drugs. The illness becomes harder to treat and the related health problems, such as organ disease, become worse.[632]

Drugs change the brain's communications system and impact the brain's normal chemical makeup. They can mimic the brain's natural chemical messengers and/or they can over stimulate the brain's natural reward

[630] Volkow, N. D., Wang, G. J., Telang, F., Fowler, J. S., Logan, J., Childress,4 A.R. et al. (2006) Cocaine Cues and Dopamine in Dorsal Striatum: Mechanism of Craving in Cocaine Addiction. *The Journal of Neuroscience*, June 14, 2006, *26*(24),6583-6588. doi:10.1523/JNEUROSCI.1544-06.2006

[631] Bechara, A. (2005) Decision making, impulse control and loss of willpower to resist drugs: A neurocognitive perspective. *Nature Neuroscience*, *8*, 1458-63.

[632] Nestler, E. J., & R. C. Malenka (2004) The addicted brain. *Scientific American*. Retrieved from: http://www.scientificamerican.com/article.cfm?id=the-addicted-brain

system.[633] For example, marijuana and heroin are drugs that share a similar structure to neurotransmitters. Because of this, marijuana and heroin can "fool" the brain's chemical receptors and cause nerve cells to send abnormal messages.

Other drugs, such as cocaine or methamphetamine, cause nerve cells to over-release natural neurotransmitters and prevent the brain from recycling these natural brain chemicals. This causes an unusually greater message to be carried, and in the end, it changes normal brain communication.[634]

When a person feeds the addiction repeatedly, over time the brain regulatory system will react to the surge in dopamine by decreasing the number of receptors on the surface of target cells, making the cells less sensitive to the dopamine. This is called "down regulation". With fewer dopamine receptors in the circuit, the reward is lessened. The drug, or sexual encounter, working longer hours or creating more chaos in their lives does not work as well as it once did and the addict is compelled to keep raising the levels in an attempt to regain the initial effect. [635] The tolerance to the drug or action is particularly dangerous, as it almost inevitably leads to a downward spiral in health.

---

[633] National Institute on Drug Abuse (2010) NIDA Info Facts: Stimulant ADHD Medications —Methylphenidate and Amphetamines. Retrieved from: http://www.drugabuse.gov/infofacts/ADHD.html

[634] Boeree, G. (2009) Neurotransmitters. Retrieved from: http://webspace.ship.edu/cgboer/genpsyneurotransmitters.html

[635] National Institute on Drug Abuse (2010a) Addiction: Drugs, Brains, and Behavior — The Science of Addiction. Retrieved from:: http://www.drugabuse.gov/scienceofaddiction/

Symptoms of addiction include:

- tolerance, or the development of resistance, to the effects of the addictive substance or activity over time
- withdrawal, a painful or unpleasant physical response when the substance or activity is withheld

It has been found that people with addictive predispositions have a lack of specific brainwave activity in the alpha frequencies. In other words, they have trouble relaxing and may feel constantly anxious and tense when not feeding their addiction.[636] This pattern can also be seen in children of alcoholics (even those who do not drink). This produces an abundance of "mental chatter." For this reason, addicts have a hard time quieting their minds. Many times these individuals use alcohol and drugs to self-soothe or slow down their brainwaves artificially. This could explain why those with addition issues also typically suffer from anxiety.

The opposite pattern can also be seen in people with addictions. Too many slow beta brainwaves can make it difficult to focus and pay attention. People with attentional problems such as ADHD have this pattern.[637] Adults with ADHD often learn to self-medicate with legal substances such as coffee and

---

[636] Collins, A. (2009) Neurofeedback for Addictions: The State of the Science. ISNR. Retrieved from:
http://www.isnr.org/information/addiction.cfm
[637] Collins, A. (2009) Neurofeedback for Addictions: The State of the Science. ISNR. Retrieved from:
http://www.isnr.org/information/addiction.cfm

cigarettes. Children and others use stimulant drugs to speed up their brainwaves and help them focus.

Other physical, social and psychological effects must also be addressed. An important aspect of addiction is cravings. Our brains are hardwired to pursue natural rewards such as food and sex because of their critical part in survival. The cravings for drugs and alcohol activate the same circuits in the brain and can be even greater than for food and sex.[638]

Food addiction is a contemporary term used to describe a pathological disorder: the compulsive, excessive craving for and consumption of food. This condition is not only manifested by the abnormal intake of food, but the intake and craving for foods that arc, in themoclvcs, harmful to the individual. While society and the medical profession have readily understood alcoholism and drug abuse, it is only in recent years that there is an equal acceptance of the fact that persons may be addicted to food in the same way. When any substance is taken into the body regardless of its potential for harm or in excess of need, that substance is said to be abused. Individuals who abuse substances in such a way are addicts; these persons become physiologically and mentally dependent upon certain substances, in this case food. This lack of control is the result of changes in the brain.

---

[638] Childress, A.R. (2010) Let's Talk About Craving. HBO online. Retrieved from: http://www.hbo.com/addiction/understanding_addiction/13_craving.html

These physical changes, in turn, cause behavioral changes.[639]

All drugs of abuse—nicotine, cocaine, marijuana, and others—affect the brain's "reward" circuit. Normally, the reward circuit responds to pleasurable experiences by releasing the neurotransmitter dopamine, which creates feelings of pleasure, and tells the brain that this is something important-pay attention and remember. Drugs hijack this system, causing unusually large amounts of dopamine to flood the system. Sometimes, this lasts for a long time compared to what happens when a natural reward stimulates dopamine. This flood of dopamine is what causes the "high" or euphoria associated with drug abuse.[640]

## THE REWARD SYSTEM

The reward system of the brain is centered in the limbic system. This area is known for its ability to monitor internal homeostasis, to mediate learning and memory and to experience emotion.[641] It includes the hypothalamus, amygdala, hippocampus, septal nuclei, and anterior cingulate gyrus. Also important to this system is the limbic striatum, which includes the

---

[639] Katherine, A. (1996) Anatomy of a Food Addiction: The Brain Chemistry of Overeating. Carlsbad, CA: Gurze Books.
[640] Hyman, S. E. & Malenka, R.C. (2001) Addiction and the brain: the neurobiology of compulsion and its persistence. *Nat Rev Neurosci*; 2: 695-703
[641] Lowinson, J. H., Ruiz, P., Millman, R. B. & Langrod, J. G., eds. (1997) *Substance abuse: A comprehensive textbook, 3rd edition*. Williams and Wilkins.

nucleus accumbens, ventral caudate nucleus and the putamen.[642]

## THE INSULA

In the past few years new information on addiction has surfaced from the neuroscientific community about the importance of a long-neglected region of the brain called the insula.[643],[644] As we saw in Chapter 2, this region can be seen in both hemispheres of the cerebral cortex, one on each side, and is actually considered part of the limbic system. It has been found to be crucial for social emotions such as lust, love, disgust, hate, gratitude, guilt, empathy, resentment, self-confidence and embarrassment just to name a few.

The insula also communicates with the rest of the body through receptors in the skin and the organs. It reacts to the sensations and sends the information to other parts of the brain. It allows us to feel empathy and even to respond emotionally to music. However, the insula also responds to the body's hunger, and even to cravings. It triggers us to eat just one more bite, smoke just one more cigarette, or to consume just one more line of cocaine.[645]

---

[642] Koob, G. F. & LeMoal, M. (2006) *Neurobiology of addiction*. Elsevier Academic.

[643] Chen, Y., Dammers, J., Boers, F., Leiberg, S., Edgar, J. C., et al. (2009)The temporal dynamics of insula activity to disgust and happy facial expressions: A magnetoencephalography study. *Neuroimage, 2009* (47), 1921–1928.

[644] Taylor, K.S., Seminowicz, D.A. & Davis, K.D. (2009) Two systems of resting state connectivity between the insula and cingulate cortex. *Human Brain Mapping. 30*(9), 2731–2745.

[645] Naqvi, N. H. et. al (2007) Damage to the insula disrupts addiction to cigarette smoking. *Science , 315*,531 – 534.

In humans as well as apes, the insula has made huge evolutionary expansion in its frontal regions, especially on the right side.[646] The right anterior insula is associated with determining and selecting a "risky" over "safe" response as well as choosing the degree of harm avoidance necessary when punishment is associated with an activity. Damage to this area of the brain can create apathy, a lack of libido, even the inability to distinguish between fresh and rotten food. Although the reward area of the brain is triggered when an addict receives another dose, or a smoker smells tobacco, it's the insula-created craving that makes it so difficult to stop being addicted. This makes the Insula a very important part of the brain for addiction retraining.

Several studies have shown that neurofeedback is effective in regaining control over this area and so the cravings of addiction.[647]

## How can it be helped?

Although addiction is a chronic disease, it is treatable. Neurotherapy allows the addict to control his own brain without drugs and alcohol. In this way, addictions can be overcome without having to suffer a lifetime of struggle and craving. Neurotherapy can help break undesirable established mental or behavioral patterns.

---

[646] Augustine, J. R. (1996) Circuitry and functional aspects of the insular lobe in primates including humans. *Brain Research Reviews, 1996* (22), 229–244.

[647] Caria, A., Veit, R., Sitaram, R., Lotze, M., Weiskopf , N., Grodd , W., et al. (2007) Regulation of anterior insular cortex activity using real-time fMRI. *Neuroimage, 15*, 1238–1246.

It can help break the cycles by providing reinforcement for 'normal' function. [648],[649]

Clinical studies show that neurotherapy can

- Reduce stress and excessive tension
- Increase relaxation and cognitive awareness
- Improve the ability to recover
- Reduce the frequency of migraines, headaches, insomnia, anxiety and depression related to withdrawal
- Help recover long- and short-term memory
- Increase iq performance
- Increase the ability to focus and concentrate
- Decrease fatigue and stress
- Improve self-confidence & self-worth
- Improve decision making and problem solving

One function of neurotherapy is to stimulate and release neurotransmitters such as dopamine, serotonin, acetylcholine, norepinephrine, and endorphins. Endorphins have a morphine-like pain-relieving effect that lowers pain intensity.[650] Endorphins reduce depression and aid emotional

[648] Huang, T. & Charyton, C. (2008) A Comprehensive Review of the Psychological Effects of Brainwave Entrainment. *Alternative Therapies in Health and Medicine, 14*, 5.

[649] Lingford-Hughes, A. & Nutt, D .(2003) Neurobiology of addiction and implications for treatment. *Br J Psychiatry, 182*, 97-100.

[650] Collins, A. (2009) Neurofeedback for Addictions: The State of the Science. ISNR. Retrieved from:
http://www.isnr.org/information/addiction.cfm

stability, allowing a calmer, more restful approach to life. People who experience neurotherapy often may find that they no longer have the cravings for drugs or alcohol to stay calm. Even those who have been dependent on drugs for years can become drug-free.

## JILL'S STORY

*Jill was diagnosed with depression at the age of 14. When she came into our office she had been on drugs for 10 years. Her list of then-current drugs included:*

- *Topamax-for migraines*
- *Dexedrine-for ADD symptoms*
- *Cytomel-for thyroid*
- *Abilify -as an add-on treatment for depression, mania and*
- *schizophrenia*
- *Zoloft-for anxiety and depression*
- *Risperdol-for schizophrenia and symptoms of bipolar*
- *disorder*
- *Lexapro-for depression and generalized anxiety disorder*

*When she first arrived, her manner was very quiet and spacey. It seemed as if she did everything in slow motion. We completed an initial assessment and found her inattention to be very high and her brain speed very slow. She was extremely depressed answering "yes" to all Depression Scale questions including, "Do you think your situation is hopeless?"*

*When we looked at the oxygen levels in her forebrain, both sides had very low baselines. However, her right side was not able to utilize the oxygen as well as the left.*

*On the right she was also unable to increase her oxygen intake over a period of four minutes.*

*Her medical evaluation revealed that she had deficiencies in vitamin D-3 and B-12, excessive body inflammation and a very low thyroid level. She had slight elevations of mercury, bismuth and uranium in her fecal heavy metals tests. Her urinary heavy metals test revealed that the levels of lead and mercury were elevated.*

*Her physician recommended that she detoxify from her medications before a clear picture could be determined regarding possible supplements. Vitamin C was administered intravenously to help with any withdrawal symptoms. Vitamin B-12 and Folic Acid were added to the IV for methylation support and vitamin D-3 was added to help with depression. Jill decided to "white knuckle" her withdrawal even though Abilify has a washout period of 30 days.*

*We started with neurotherapy to assist her in relieving her depression and to help stabilize her brain so that she could eliminate the drugs. We trained at Fp1, Fp2 and Af8 to help with depression, anxiety and memory. We used a calming audio/visual entrainment setting at 7.8 Hz, neuromotor skills and cognitive training.*

*After three sessions her mother reported that "...her behavior has become bizarre—occasional friendly moments, but mostly shouting and throwing things. Perseverating about things—nothing in the house has any privacy, she is tearing through the closets, leaves stuff on the floor that she is knocking off the shelves. She is extremely up-tight, can't figure out what to wear,* clothes are just everywhere." Her mother saw her getting worse and displaying great anger. Her physician opined that the likely cause of these symptoms was the anxiety and physical withdrawal from medication.

As we continued therapy, Jill would go through periods of cold sweats and shaking, headaches and body aches. She commented as she was weaning herself from Dexedrine that it felt just like withdrawing from cocaine. She craved Dexedrine more intensely than any of the other medications. Nevertheless, she persevered. After the next five sessions she started to feel better.

By the end of the neurotherapy sessions, she was completely off all of her medications and no longer felt depressed. Her final note to us was poignant and gratifying:

---

"From the bottom of my heart, thank you. Not only for this, but for helping me regain my life and live again. I think about the state of being I was in when I first came to see you and where I am now and will continue to improve and I am very grateful for all your help. I had no hope and you helped me regain that."

---

One interesting aspect of Jill's case was that she had apparently stopped growing emotionally at age 14 when she started taking the prescribed drugs. Her mother now noticed all of the behaviors of a teen-aged girl. Over the period of three or four months following the *neurotherapy she started to "catch up" with those of her age group. By the time she was done she was a happy, mature 24-year-old woman.*

# CHAPTER 17
# THE BRAIN AND
# PEAK
# PERFORMANCE

In this book we have discussed many issues common amongst our patients. However anyone can benefit from brain training. For those with "well brains", their goal might be to have better athletic skills, academic success or corporate prowess. Peak Performance is a term we hear a lot today. It refers to the ability to alter your state of mind voluntarily in order to most effectively meet any challenge. Studies of successful athletes have shown that, in addition to a high level of skill, they share the characteristics of:

- Control over body and mind states
- A high level of focused concentration

Anyone who has played a sport knows that competition can create an intense emotional response. However for your performance to be consistent, you must first be able to manage that emotional surge and use it to your advantage instead of letting it control you.

Stress from everyday life can also affect your game. Work, finances, or family matters can take a toll, making it much more difficult to relax and focus during competition. Even balancing full-time employment or education combined with the demands of elite competition can be overwhelming. So it stands to reason that those who are able to effectively regulate emotions such as fear, mind chatter, excitement, lethargy and sluggishness, have an advantage over those that can't.

Though the term "peak performance" could apply to a number of different areas of self-improvement, one thing is clear – having peak performance implies that you are operating at the top of your game.

## How to Get the Edge

If you watch professional sports you'll notice that the difference in actual scores between high-ranking athletes and those with the rest of the pack is usually very small. Meaning in most cases, it doesn't take much to go from number 3 to number 1. However, the biomechanics of the game can only take you so far. After all, every successful athlete trains hard. But winning athletes know that training the body is only the first step in winning competitions. They know training the brain is as important, maybe even more so, than the rigorous physical exercise and training done to improve physical skill. The ability to control the mind as well as the body allows an athlete to consistently perform at their highest level of competency.

In the past, sports psychologists have used talk therapy, visualization techniques and hypnosis to try and help athletes with these issues. More recently neurotherapy has come to light as a way to give the athlete a tool to discipline the brain just as they have disciplined the physical body. It turns out it is less about visualizing the ball going into a hole, or the perfect swing, it is actually about the larger picture. It's about teaching the individual mental discipline to control their entire life rather than the act of visualizing an effective shot. With this knowledge, it is amazing that training the brain is seldom considered in athletics. Virtually all the emphasis is placed on physical skills.

Neurotherapy training is an effective approach for athletes desiring to improve their performance. It focuses on training the brain to relax under pressure, to get and stay in the zone and shut out mental chatter that distracts you from your goal. These mental skills allow you to mentally and physically engage in the game without any emotional or mental interference, allowing you to perform at your best every time.

To play a game effectively, a flexible state of mind is at the core. This means the ability to change mental states easily and appropriately for each move. An athlete is required to quickly visually process the layout of the course and plan moves spatially according to distance, direction, as well as environmental elements such as wind and terrain. They need to recognize their own body in space and position themselves for their ultimate performance. Then effortlessly, they must shift into a relaxed calm; to block out interference from sounds in the environment as well as nervous tension and chatter within their own mind. This calm helps the brain and body act together smoothly making the long-practiced move automatic and true. Afterwards, the athlete must once again change mental gears to process the results and prepare for the challenge. Finally, the athlete must be able to remain calm and relaxed to repeat this method for each complex maneuver without becoming overtired, frustrated or angry. This type of training cannot be mastered with biomechanics training. This is something above and beyond the usual. It provides you with that "something extra" that takes your performance into the next level.

In recent years, Peak Performance neurotherapy techniques have emerged to help the athlete enhance their ability to reduce anxiety and get into "the zone". This became newsworthy in 2006 when the Italian soccer team discovered when they focused on retraining their thinking by using neurofeedback, along with guided imagery and other cognitive restructuring techniques, they won the World Cup. These techniques teach the brain to improve its performance. They allow the athlete to improve concentration, inconsistent play, frustration and other problems that keep them from reaching their full athletic potential. Neurotherapy also helps reduce emotions and mental chatter that obstruct peak performance. It allows athletes to increase their mental acuity, relaxation and mental flexibility, gain clarity, resist outside pressures and sustain that important mental edge.

## IS PEAK PERFORMANCE LIMITED TO SPORTS?

In this chapter we focus on athletes, but just like sports, other things in life can be influenced by improved brain performance. Business people have the same issues as athletes. Concerns over the economy, job loss, money issues and poor sleep, stress and self-doubt can all spiral down into a mindset which is very hard to reverse. You start to ruminate about your poor performance, how bad you are such as, "I don't feel good" or "I'm never going to be a success. Everything is bad." In fact, just like we saw in Chapter 14, those thoughts could be at the very root of the problem.

After all, a business person is competing in a high stress corporate world. An employer is always striving to improve the performance and creativity of their employees. Neurotherapy can help them:

- Improve cognitive function—think better and smarter
- *Lower stress*—tap into that relaxation vein whenever needed
- *Increase mental flexibility*—always be able to respond to a challenge quickly and accurately
- *Increase memory*—keep those important facts always on tap

Even Human Resources Departments can implement neurotherapy to provide these benefits to both the company and its employees. According to the American Heart Association, The high direct medical care and indirect costs of cardiovascular disease due to stress-related illness was $450 billion in 2010 and projected to rise to over $1 trillion a year by 2030. [651] It is estimated that 70% of health care costs are preventable. Therefore, having a less stressful environment and a more productive work force cuts down on absenteeism and insurance costs for the employer.

---

[651] American Heart Association (2011) Value of Primordial and Primary Prevention for Cardiovascular Disease : A Policy Statement From the American Heart Association. *Circulation.* Retrieved from http://circ.ahajournals.org/content/early/2011/07/25/CIR.0b013e318 2285a81.full.pdf

Costs of lost productivity are substantial and have been studied extensively. Distinct subcategories of productivity exist, for example, absenteeism, or reduced productivity because the person is absent from work for health reasons, and decreased productivity while at work. Other factors include premature mortality, impaired quality of life, increased rates of disability benefit payments, and increased medical care costs.

Neurotherapy can help reduce stress, depression and anxiety making life more manageable. This translates into happier and healthier employees.

How does our BrainAdvantage system work? It provides you with more information about your brain and body than your normal senses can provide. Tools to enhance brain activity and promote better function, help communication between both hemispheres of the brain to help them synchronize more efficiently and tools to relax the brain and help teach the mind to easily change into its best relaxed state. Other tools for eye convergence, auditory and visual processing as well as cognitive improvement are available.

But don't confuse BrainAdvantage with other brain training programs. BrainAdvantage is different. We know that the brain and body are connected. The brain cannot be "fixed" apart from the rest. We look at the whole body and balance everything for better brain function. We know that one size doesn't fit all and a single therapy doesn't work for everyone. Therefore we provide an individualized, integrated system of several technologies to help each client maximize the benefit they receive from the program.

# Epilogue

By the time you read this, BrainAdvantage will have been researching and treating patients for more than ten years. We have had offices in Scottsdale, Arizona, San Clemente, California and Hilton Head Island, South Carolina. Our patients have come from the locales around our offices and from around the country, the continent, and the world. We have helped patients from Canada, Europe, China, and across the Midwestern United States, where we have no offices.

Over the years, we have treated patients aged three to 92 and with brain issues from Traumatic Brain Injury to Autism Spectrum Disorder to Obsessive-Compulsive Disorder. And we have helped virtually every patient. The stories you have read in this book are all based on real patients who received real help through our offices. The success is real and the patients have retained that success after the end of their treatment protocols.

It is impossible to describe how gratifying it has been to have designed The BrainAdvantage System and then to see it in action helping people. We see them stop taking drugs, learn control over their brain processes and gain in brain function in a variety of ways. When a mother tells us, "You have given my son back to me," or a little girl volunteers, "This is the start of my new life," our hearts are full.

BrainAdvantage has seen success on both coasts. The population around our Hilton Head Island office has let us hone our services to seniors with satisfying results. Moreover, we have been able to prove that our system can be delivered through a range of channels, letting us broaden our delivery approach while still maintaining the appropriate level of supervision and safety.

As we have accumulated patient success after success, we have heard interesting comments from our patients at the close of their course of therapy. As we treat them for anxiety and depression, for example, they might find that they are better able to compete on the motorcycle track or to play Bach with more fluidity. Video gamers report that everything seems to slow for them and they are able to improve their scores in games they could never beat before. Divers are able to do more complex dives and score higher in the dives they already performed. In short, we had been helping their whole brain performance, not just helping with specific areas.

As a result of these patient reports, we began extending our services to those with well brains, with the express goal of helping athletes improve their performances. Our in-house research showed that some of the same tools that are a part of our BrainAdvantage System can also help athletes "get in the zone" and compete with more success. With this in mind, we have been designing a new BrainAdvantage Peak Performance System.

It is not just athletic performance that has benefited from the BrainAdvantage System. We have had businesspeople seeing us for anxiety issues report that after the completion of their course of treatment, they are better able to focus at work tasks and return to work more quickly when distracted. They credit our system for these gains.

The BrainAdvantage experience has been a blessing for us and for our patients. We have strived to make it the most pleasant and supportive experience available. No needles, no sticky electrodes, beautiful music, enticing videos, calming or stimulating brain wave entrainment —these are all parts of what our patients enjoy. In fact, we have had more than one young patient intentionally "fail" his ending assessment so that he can continue to come to our office for treatment. Of course, we find a reason for them to continue-for free, if circumstances merit. We love these patients and they seem to love us, as well.

# About the Author

DR. STEPHANIE REESE has been researching and working in the neurotherapy field for more than a decade. She has a Ph.D. in Cognitive Science and Technologies and is co-founder of BrainAdvantage, LLC.

Her career has spanned diverse fields from twenty years as a radiologic technologist to educator, artist, and author of several books.

Dr. Reese was the driving force behind the founding of BrainAdvantage and served as its Chief Science Officer. Her understanding of the needs of children with ADHD guided the development of The BrainAdvantage System and its success at the heart of the company's national operations.

Dr. Reese lives in Mukilteo, Washington. She has four children, nine grandchildren, and four opinionated dogs.

Made in the USA
Las Vegas, NV
30 March 2022

46557001R10246